Mental Health Services for Vulnerable Children and Young People

More than half of children either in foster care, or adopted from care in the developed world, have a measurable need for mental health services, while up to one quarter present with complex and severe trauma- and attachment-related psychological disorders. This book outlines how services can effectively detect, prevent and treat mental health difficulties in this vulnerable population.

Responding to increasing evidence that standard child and adolescent mental health services are poorly matched to the mental health service needs of children and young people who have been in foster care, this book provides expert guidance on the design of specialised services. The first part provides an overview of these children's mental health needs, their use of mental health services and what is known about the effectiveness of mental health interventions provided to them. The second part presents some recent innovations in mental health service delivery, concentrating on advances in clinical and developmental assessment and treatment. The final part confronts the challenges for delivering effective mental health services in this area.

This is the definitive international reference for the design of specialised mental health services for children and young people in care and those adopted from care. It is invaluable reading for health and social care professionals working with this population and academics with an interest in child and adolescent mental health from a range of disciplines, including social work, nursing and psychology.

Michael Tarren-Sweeney is a Clinical Psychologist, Epidemiologist and Child Developmental Theorist. He is Associate Professor of Child and Family Psychology at Canterbury University in New Zealand (where he teaches postgraduate psychology trainees through to board registration), as well as a Consultant Clinical Psychologist for government and charitable children's agencies in Australia.

Arlene Vetere is Professor of Clinical Psychology and Deputy Director of the PsychD in clinical psychology at Surrey University, UK. She is Professor of Family Therapy and Systemic Practice at Diakonhjemmet University College, Oslo, Norway. She is a UKCP Registered Systemic Psychotherapist and HCPC Registered Clinical Psychologist.

Routledge Advances in Health and Social Policy

New titles

Health Care Reform and Globalisation
The US, China and Europe in Comparative Perspective
Edited by Peggy Watson

Power and Welfare
Understanding Citizens' Encounters with State Welfare
Nanna Mik-Meyer and Kaspar Villadsen

International Perspectives on Elder Abuse
Amanda Phelan

Mental Health Services for Vulnerable Children and Young People
Supporting children who are, or have been, in foster care
Michael Tarren-Sweeney and Arlene Vetere

Forthcoming titles

M-Health in Developing Countries
Design and Implementation Perspectives on Using Mobiles in Healthcare
Arul Chib

Alcohol Policy in Europe
Delivering the WHO Ideal?
Shane Butler, Karen Elmeland and Betsy Thom

Mental Health Services for Vulnerable Children and Young People

Supporting children who are, or have been, in foster care

Edited by
Michael Tarren-Sweeney and
Arlene Vetere

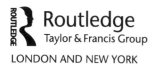

LONDON AND NEW YORK

First published 2014
by Routledge

Published 2014 by Routledge
2 Park Square, Milton Park, Abingdon, Oxfordshire OX14 4RN

Simultaneously published in the USA and Canada
by Routledge
711 Third Avenue, New York, NY 10017

Routledge is an imprint of the Taylor and Francis Group, an informa business

First issued in paperback 2015

© 2014 selection and editorial material, Michael Tarren-Sweeney and Arlene Vetere; individual chapters, the contributors

The right of the editor to be identified as the author of the editorial material, and of the authors for their individual chapters, has been asserted in accordance with sections 77 and 78 of the Copyright, Designs and Patents Act 1988.

All rights reserved. No part of this book may be reprinted or reproduced or utilised in any form or by any electronic, mechanical, or other means, now known or hereafter invented, including photocopying and recording, or in any information storage or retrieval system, without permission in writing from the publishers.

Trademark notice: Product or corporate names may be trademarks or registered trademarks, and are used only for identification and explanation without intent to infringe.

British Library Cataloguing in Publication Data
A catalogue record for this book is available from the British Library

Library of Congress Cataloging in Publication Data
Mental health services for vulnerable children and young people : supporting children who are, or have been, in foster care / edited by Michael Tarren-Sweeney and Arlene Vetere.
 p.; cm. – (Routledge advances in health and social policy)
Includes bibliographical references.
I. Tarren-Sweeney, Michael. II. Vetere, Arlene. III. Series: Routledge advances in health and social policy.
[DNLM: 1. Mental Health Services. 2. Adolescent. 3. Adoption–psychology. 4. Child. 5. Foster Home Care–psychology. 6. Infant. 7. Needs Assessment. WM 30.1]
362.2083–dc23
2012050564

ISBN 978-0-415-63268-3 (hbk)
ISBN 978-1-138-96016-9 (pbk)
ISBN 978-0-203-09547-8 (ebk)

Typeset in Goudy
by Taylor and Francis Books

Contents

Contributors	vii
Foreword	xii
LORD LISTOWEL (FRANCIS HARE)	

PART I
Overview 1

1 Establishing the need for mental health services for children and young people in care, and those who are subsequently adopted 3
MICHAEL TARREN-SWEENEY AND ARLENE VETERE

2 The benefits of outpatient mental health services for children in long-term foster care 21
JENNIFER BELLAMY, GEETHA GOPALAN AND DORIAN TRAUBE

3 Our twenty-first century quest: Locating effective mental health interventions for children and young people in care, and those adopted from care 37
MICHAEL TARREN-SWEENEY

PART II
Recent innovations in mental health service delivery 59

4 Enhancing adoptive parenting: From a trial of effectiveness to translation 61
ALAN RUSHTON

5 The 'Spirit of New Orleans': Translating a model of intervention with maltreated children and their families for the Glasgow context 83
HELEN MINNIS, GRAHAM BRYCE, LOUISE PHIN AND PHILIP WILSON

vi Contents

6 Social-emotional screening and intervention for 0–4-year-old children entering care   99
CAROL HARDY AND ELIZABETH MURPHY

7 Using an attachment narrative approach with families where the children are looked after or adopted   119
RUDI DALLOS AND ANNIE DALLOS

PART III
Designing specialised mental health services for children in care, and those adopted from care   139

8 Ten years later: The experience of a CAMHS service for children in care   141
MEGAN CHAMBERS

9 Multi-agency and specialist working to meet the mental health needs of children in care and adopted   161
KIM S. GOLDING

10 Some reflections on the use of psychiatric diagnosis in the looked after or 'in care' child population   180
MARGARET DEJONG

11 The making and breaking of relationships: Organisational and clinical questions in establishing a family life for looked after children   194
JOHN SIMMONDS

12 Principles for the design of mental health services for children and young people in care, and those adopted from care   210
MICHAEL TARREN-SWEENEY

Index   225

Contributors

Editors

Michael Tarren-Sweeney is a clinical psychologist, epidemiologist and child developmental theorist. He is associate professor of Child and Family Psychology at Canterbury University in New Zealand (where he teaches postgraduate psychology trainees through to board registration), as well as a consultant clinical psychologist for government and charitable children's agencies in Australia. His life's work has focused on the nature and causes of mental ill-health experienced by children and young people in care, and the implications this has for social care policy and practice, and for mental health services. Michael recently completed the Children in Care study – a decade-long, population study of the mental health and psychosocial development of children in foster and kinship care. As part of this work, he developed the Assessment Checklist series of instruments (ACC, ACA, ACC+, BAC-C, BAC-A) to measure a range of mental health difficulties experienced among children and adolescents in care (see www.childpsych.org.uk). Michael is presently working on a developmental theory of the psychosocial effects of impermanent care, to be tested in a cross-national, longitudinal effects study.

Arlene Vetere is professor of clinical psychology and deputy director of the PsychD in Clinical psychology at Surrey University, UK. She is professor of family therapy and systemic practice at Diakonhjemmet University College, Oslo, Norway. She is a UKCP registered systemic psychotherapist and HCPC registered clinical psychologist. This integration is the foundation for her work with family violence, where she takes a particular interest in the effects of exposure to interpersonal violence on psychological development across the lifespan.

Chapter authors

Jennifer Bellamy is an assistant professor at the School of Social Service Administration (SSA) at the University of Chicago. At SSA she teaches courses in clinical social work practice and integrating research evidence into practice. She completed her doctoral training at the Columbia University School of Social Work in 2006 and postdoctoral training at the George Warren Brown School of Social Work at Washington University in Saint Louis. Her current research interests include mental health services for families involved in or at risk of involvement in child welfare, the engagement of fathers in child and family services, and evidence-based practice. She has published extensively in the area of evidence-based social work practice and is currently engaged in research projects focused on adaptations to evidence-based parenting interventions, including home visiting and parent training, to increase fathers' engagement and reduce the risk of child maltreatment.

Graham Bryce is a child and adolescent psychiatrist with a long interest in improving access to appropriate mental health services for children. He led the Scottish CAMH Needs Assessment and has served as an advisor to Scottish Government. He works in a clinical team dedicated to developing and providing mental health services for children who are looked after in local authority care.

Megan Chambers is a child and adolescent psychiatrist who has worked in a range of CAMHS as both a clinician and in leadership roles. She is currently the Director of Redbank House, an in-patient and day-patient psychiatric hospital in Western Sydney with programmes for children and young people from birth to 18 years. For the past 12 years she has had a particular interest in the development of services and service delivery models for children in out of home care, and the functioning of effective partnerships which facilitate these.

Annie Dallos is a registered children and families Social Worker and UKCP registered Family Therapist. Annie works for a community-based early intervention Family Therapy service in Plymouth and has an independent practice. She is a training provider and systemic supervisor for local authority social care staff. She has a particular interest in working therapeutically with looked after children in permanent placements and their carers.

Rudi Dallos is professor and research director on the Doctorate in Clinical Psychology Training Programme at the University of Plymouth (UK). He has been co-editor of the journal *Clinical Child Psychology and Psychiatry* and has conducted research and published in the area of systemic family therapy and attachment. His books include: 'An Introduction to Family Therapy', 'Attachment Narrative Therapy' and 'Systemic Therapy and Attachment Narratives'.

Margaret DeJong is a consultant child and adolescent psychiatrist and head of the Department of Child and Adolescent Mental Health at Great Ormond Street Hospital for Children as well as Honorary Senior

Lecturer at the Institute of Child Health, University College London. She runs the Parenting and Child Service, an assessment and therapeutic service for children with a background of abuse, neglect and trauma. This includes multidisciplinary expert witness work in complex child protection cases, in which she has many years of experience. She has a background in general CAMHS and paediatric liaison work, a diploma in advanced family therapy from the Tavistock Clinic and a longstanding interest in parenting difficulties relating to child protection issues. She has published in the field of maltreatment.

Kim S. Golding is a clinical psychologist with a longstanding interest in collaborating with parents to develop their parenting skills tailored to the particular needs of the children they are caring for. She has a special interest in supporting foster carers and adoptive parents. Kim was involved in the setting up and evaluation of an inter-agency project in Worcestershire, UK. This team is now part of the Integrated Service for Looked After and Adopted Children (ISL). She has carried out research exploring a consultation model for foster carers and the professional network around a child and has been involved in an evaluation of the Fostering Attachments Group for foster and adoptive parents. Kim is author of 'Nurturing Attachments' and co-author of 'Thinking Psychologically About Children who are Looked After and Adopted' and 'Creating Loving Attachments'.

Geetha Gopalan is a post-doctoral fellow at the New York University Silver School of Social Work, and is affiliated with the McSilver Institute for Poverty Policy and Research. She is currently funded through the National Institute of Mental Health (NIMH: F32MH090614) through a National Research Science Award post-doctoral fellowship. Dr Gopalan is also an investigator with the Implementation Research Institute (IRI), at the George Warren Brown School of Social Work, Washington University in St. Louis; through an award from the National Institute of Mental Health (R25 MH080916-01A2) and the Department of Veterans Affairs, Health Services Research & Development Service, Quality Enhancement Research Initiative (QUERI). Dr Gopalan's research interests involve designing, implementing and testing family-level interventions to improve youth mental health and reduce youth risk behaviour, particularly for families with intensive service involvement and extreme psychosocial needs (such as those involved in the child welfare system).

Carol Hardy is a clinical specialist in a CAMH service for Children in Care in Southwark, South London. For the past 25 years her main clinical interest has focused on developing assessment and interventions with babies and primary age children along with their birth parents, foster carers or adoptive parents. Her clinical work has been in teams based in the inner city, working with high-risk and vulnerable populations. She has provided teaching to a wide variety of professionals and carers along with the development of specific training programmes. In the past two years she developed and delivered the screening study described in this book with the collaboration of colleagues across services/agencies.

Helen Minnis is an academic child and adolescent psychiatrist with a research and clinical interest in the difficulties associated with early maltreatment. She has published research on Reactive Attachment Disorder and also on interventions and services for children in foster care.

Elizabeth Murphy is a consultant child and adolescent psychotherapist and lead clinician at Southwark CAMHS, where she runs their Looked after Children's team. She has worked in a range of mental health services, both in-patient and community teams, and for the last 20 years has worked primarily with looked after children and their carers. In addition to having a keen interest in service and clinical developments she has participated in research. Most recently with colleagues she completed research on screening for mental health needs in looked after children aged 4–16 years and has collaborated with Carol Hardy on the project described in this book.

Louise Phin is qualified as a chartered clinical psychologist from Lancaster University in 2008 and is now working in a children and young people's mental health team in South Lanarkshire, Scotland. Working in child and family services has led to an interest in attachment-based psychotherapies, infant mental health and the promotion of mental well-being in families.

Alan Rushton spent many years as a social worker in both child and adult mental health services in the UK and in Canada. For over 25 years he was director of the MSc programme in Mental Health Social Work at the Institute of Psychiatry, King's College London where he continues as Visiting Professor. He has been engaged in follow-up studies of older, abused children adopted from care and in predictors of placement outcome. Alan has published many academic papers and recent books have included 'Adoption support services for families in difficulty', 'Enhancing adoptive parenting: a test of effectiveness' and 'Enhancing adoptive parenting: a parenting programme for use with adopters of challenging children'. He is a member of the British Chinese Adoption Study team and is a Trustee at the Post-Adoption Centre in London.

John Simmonds is director of Policy, Research and Development at the British Association for Adoption and Fostering (BAAF). Before starting at BAAF, he was head of the social work programmes at Goldsmiths College, University of London. He is a qualified social worker and has substantial experience in child protection, family placement and residential care settings. He has published widely including editing with Gillian Schofield the 'Child Placement Handbook' and 'Good Practice Guidance on Special

Guardianship', both published by BAAF. He recently completed a research project on unaccompanied asylum-seeking children in foster care with the University of York and a study of women placed 50 years ago from Hong Kong in UK adoptive families. He recently started a DFE-funded project on outcomes for children placed through Special Guardianship also with York. He is the adoptive father of two children, now adults.

Dorian Traube is an assistant professor at the University of Southern California School of Social Work. Her scholarship focuses on the behavioural health of high-risk adolescents. In this context, behavioural health refers to promoting physical and mental well-being by preventing or treating mental illness and substance abuse for high-risk populations of youth between the ages of 13 and 24. Her scholarly contributions have occurred in three topic areas: (1) the behavioural health of adolescents affected by AIDS; (2) the behavioural health of young men who have sex with men; and (3) the behavioural health of child welfare involved adolescents. These areas converge to meet her primary research agenda of translating models of behavioural risk across high-risk adolescent populations.

Philip Wilson is an academic general practitioner with an interest in early childhood mental health and in the development and evaluation of complex interventions. He recently completed a career scientist aware in infant mental health and has published papers on early identification of psychiatric problems in children.

Foreword

Lord Listowel (Francis Hare)

I am very fortunate as a cross-bench member of the House of Lords to have been involved in many issues connected to our looked after children population. This has involved extensive contact with professionals and particularly young people who have spent a number if not many years in foster or residential care. I have been privileged to chair the All Party Parliamentary Group for Looked After Children and Care Leavers, a group that regularly hears from young people about their experiences and concerns and makes strong representations to government and other stakeholders about what and what doesn't work well. I have also been fortunate to be invited to observe, discuss and reflect on these matters more directly in a wide range of settings where young people are cared for. I have no doubt that we have much to applaud in the dedication, insight and expertise of the professionals and carers who commit themselves to either arranging or directly caring for these young people 24 hours a day, 7 days a week. But that is not to say that all is well – resources are stretched, demands are high and the complexity of many of the situations young people find themselves in defy easy explanation or solution.

Mental health is a challenging concept. It often invites stigma, is something to be avoided because of the stigma and can feel like one more burden to be endured amongst many others. It cannot be surprising, however, that the factors that lead up to a young person being looked after – abuse or neglect or serious family breakdown – can lead to a range of responses – distress, anxiety or depression. It also cannot be surprising if there are other developmental challenges from learning difficulties to a range of psychological and social disorders. If we know one thing about child development, it is thoroughly embedded in a family life that is secure, enduring and stable. Family breakdown is exactly the opposite of what children need and that is the challenge for the looked after children's system – how to re-construct the child's family or how to construct a new family that has all the characteristics that we know children need. And we know for some children there will be a number of intermediate steps along the way – in temporary, sometimes specialist foster or residential care.

Identifying, naming and addressing mental health issues in this process couldn't be more important. And that is why this book couldn't be more timely. It is sensitively written by a wide range of experts, extremely detailed in unpicking the complexity of the issues, and appropriately cautious and realistic about what can be and needs to be done, in the provision of services. Above all it is humane in its overall approach. And that reflects my experience of so many of the young people I have met. They want their experiences to be acknowledged and that may mean their distress, their fears and their anxieties. But in acknowledging any of this, they need to know that professionals are above all humane, sensitive to and committed to try to move things on. They see the person in the professional and that matters a lot. Where they only see the professional, then that can be disappointing and upsetting. Finding ways of combining the personal and the professional in making relationships with young people is one of the biggest lessons I have learnt over the years and I was heartened to see that reflected in so many ways in the chapters that go to make up this valuable collection of papers.

Lord Listowel, Cross Bench Member of the House of Lords

Part I
Overview

1 Establishing the need for mental health services for children and young people in care, and those who are subsequently adopted

Michael Tarren-Sweeney and Arlene Vetere

No other groups of children and young people in the developed world are more socially or developmentally disadvantaged than children and young people who reside in court-ordered alternate care, and those who are subsequently adopted from care. Prior to entering care, they mostly endure profound social adversity, including traumatic abuse and emotional deprivation. By and large, their pre-care adversity exceeds that endured by the much larger group of maltreated children who remain in their parents' care. Following their entry into care and/or transition to adoption, these groups have to navigate a host of systemically driven assaults on their well-being and felt security. This book seeks to redress some important social and psychological manifestations of their disadvantage, including mental ill-health, emotional distress and behavioural difficulties – by disseminating the best knowledge we have on prevention and treatment of those difficulties *for these populations*, and by highlighting the present gaps in our knowledge, and the inadequacies of prevailing service models.

The idea for publishing this book came about in 2010, after we had edited a special issue of *Clinical Child Psychology and Psychiatry* (October, 2010) on the topic of mental health services for children and young people in care and those adopted from care. The special issue generated a lot of interest and discussion, particularly from clinicians working in child welfare, alternate care and adoption fields, and from people working on mental health services policy within health and social care agencies. These populations exert exceptional demands on poorly matched, generic mental health services – a dilemma that most child welfare and child mental health jurisdictions in the developed world are presently struggling with. The response to the special issue supports our belief that the provision of appropriate and sufficient mental health services for these vulnerable populations will remain a key concern for child mental health and social care agencies over the coming decades. To that end, we set out to publish a definitive international reference guide for the design of specialised mental health services for children in care (and those adopted from care) – one that is equally useful for clinicians and clinical leaders, child mental health and social care agencies, government departments and policy makers.

To make this happen, we were fortunate to enlist the assistance of some of the world's best thinkers in this field of practice and research. Advancing the well-being and psychological development of children in various types of alternate care (and reducing their felt distress) is a vocation shared by each of the book's contributors. For most contributors, this has been the focus of their life's work! Importantly, each contributor brings a mix of practitioner experience in working with these children, and considered scholarship. What communicates most forcefully from their contributions to this book is the need for a drastic reappraisal and overhaul of mental health services provided to children in care and those adopted from care.

Children and young people in the care and adoption systems

At any given time, perhaps a million children in the western world either reside in legally mandated alternate care, or have been adopted from such care. A substantially larger population encounters alternate care at some time in their childhood. Children residing in court-ordered care are collectively referred to as *looked after* children in Britain and Ireland, and as children in *out-of-home care* in North America and Australasia – although neither term satisfactorily describes the status of children in long-term alternate care. Many jurisdictions witnessed a doubling of the rate of children in care between the mid-90s and mid-2000s, which in 2005 averaged around 5 per 1000 children across western, Anglophone nations (Holzer & Bromfield, 2008). This change continues unabated in Australia, where the rate increased by 26% (from 5.8 to 7.3 per 1000) between 2007 and 2011 (Australian Institute of Health and Welfare, 2012). By comparison, there was a 9% increase (from 6 to 6.6 per 1000) in the number of children in care (including those adopted from care) in Britain over the same four-year period (Department for Education, 2011). These increases are largely accounted for by a corresponding acceleration in the detection of child maltreatment. Variations in national rates of children in care partially reflect the provision of long-term solutions such as return to birth parents, adoption from care and/or special guardianship orders. They also reflect shifting thresholds of concern, particularly as agencies are subjected to public outcries when children who are formally safeguarded by the State die through lack of proper supervision or services.

While there is considerable variation in care systems, most western jurisdictions shifted emphasis from non-family residential care to foster care through the late twentieth century, and more recently to kinship care and adoption from care. Kinship care is partly driven in Australia, New Zealand and Canada by concern for the identity and well-being of large and disproportionate numbers of indigenous children in care (see for example Lock, (1997)). In Britain and North America, adoption from care is the preferred 'permanent' outcome for children who are either unable to return to parental care, and for whom there is no suitable kinship placement. In the year ending March 2011, 3050 children in care were adopted in Britain (Department for Education, 2011), constituting a fairly small proportion of those who are eligible for adoption. Furthermore, the annual numbers of British children in care who are placed for adoption, and who are adopted, fell between 2007 and 2011 (Department for Education, 2011). This situation is contrary to public policy and permanency goals, and has prompted a recent government review of adoption in Britain. In Australasia, adoption from care is more difficult to achieve, and is thus uncommon. Any move to formalise the adoption of Australian children from care would invoke resistance because of that country's history of forcible and unjust removal of aboriginal children (the 'stolen generation'). Instead, in Australia and New Zealand early-placed children who are not restored to parental care are typically raised in quasi-adoptive foster or kinship placements. A surprisingly large number of early-placed children are retained in long-term care in England as well, as a part of more general permanency policy (Biehal, Ellison, Baker, & Sinclair, 2009; Schofield & Ward, 2008). These children are more likely to endure greater systemic threats to their 'felt security' than children adopted from care, such as the realisation of their carers' lack of custody rights, and the State's intrusion throughout their childhood (Nutt, 2006). Otherwise these groups have comparable developmental pathways, invoking similar risk for attachment- and trauma-related mental health difficulties.

Developmental underpinnings

Mental health and resilience among children in care, and those who are subsequently adopted, arise from complex, time-sensitive interactions between genotype, prenatal conditions, pre-care and in-care psychosocial conditions and events, and infant neurological development (Rutter, 2000). The social experiences that predicate entry into care represent critical developmental risks for their well-being and mental health. Foremost of these is exposure to psychological trauma, emotional deprivation and other conditions that negate opportunity for secure attachments. Children in care also encounter a number of uncommon developmental events, the most critical being the loss of their biological parents, integration into new families or non-family settings, and (for some at least) unstable placements. Developmental psychopathology models pertaining to maltreated children (Cicchetti, Toth, & Maughan, 2000) and profoundly deprived inter-country adoptees (O'Connor, Bredenkamp, Rutter, & the English and Romanian Adoptees Study Team, 1999) are thus only partially valid for children in care, as there are both commonalities and differences in their experience. Conversely, there is considerable commonality in the developmental pathways of children raised in long-term foster care and children who are subsequently adopted from care.

Risk studies of children in care have identified several predictors of mental health difficulties and other negative outcomes, notably older age at entry into care, placement instability, perceived placement insecurity, and intellectual disability (Delfabbro & Barber, 2003; Tarren-Sweeney, 2008c). Younger age at entry into family-type (i.e. foster and kinship) care appears to be protective for subsequent mental health (Fanshel & Shinn, 1978; Tarren-Sweeney, 2008c), while early placement in residential care is harmful (Johnson, Browne, & Hamilton-Giachritsis, 2006). These findings can be interpreted in terms of 'cumulative adversity' and 'attachment' models. Whereas a single harmful event may have life-altering developmental consequences for children at large, the impact of individual events is tempered among children exposed to chronic and multiple adversities. A number of researchers have reported that broad indicators of exposure to adversity and to other risk factors account for a greater proportion of the variance in children's mental health, than exposure to specific types or single instances of harm (Fergusson & Lynskey, 1996; Rutter, 1999). For instance, it has been shown that length of exposure to maltreatment and the number of maltreatment events are stronger predictors than the type of harm encountered by children (Tarren-Sweeney, 2008c; Zeanah, Boris, & Larrieu, 1997). Similarly, among children with multiple genetic vulnerabilities, individual genetic risks account for small proportions of the variance in their mental health (Plomin, DeFries, & McClearn, 1997).

Age at entry into care also has significance in terms of attachment quality, and related emotional and neurological development. Children who are emotionally deprived and/or abused, are likely to develop insecure or disorganised attachments to their caregivers, or worse, manifest attachment disorder behaviours (Howe & Fearnley, 2003; Newman & Mares, 2007; O'Connor & Zeanah, 2003). Such difficulties are in turn moderately correlated with the presence of behavioural and emotional problems (Marcus, 1991). While a number of studies have articulated differences in the attachment behaviours of abused versus neglected children (Crittenden & Ainsworth, 1989), this is an artificial distinction for children in care. In addition to abuse and neglect, other pre-care experiences account for the development of attachment difficulties among such children. Attachment theory would predict that the therapeutic potential of alternate care and adoption should vary according to: 1. the characteristics of children's attachment systems prior to entering care; and 2. carer sensitivity and ability to provide a 'secure base' following entry into care (Bowlby, 1988; Schofield, 2002). Some children are cared for by a succession of strangers for lengthy periods (sometimes extending to weeks or months). Some endure successive losses, both prior to and following entry into care, resulting in grief, confusion and insecurity. For example, a child might reside with her birth mother to age 18 months, then with her grandmother to age 30 months, then back to her mother, and so on. In this scenario, the child resides long enough with her mother, and thence with her grandmother, to become successively attached to each caregiver. But her relationships are rendered insecure upon losing them.

Regardless of prior conditions, the attachment systems of infants who enter foster care are found to be responsive to changes in parenting style

(Dozier, Stovall, Albus, & Bates, 2001; Steele, Hodges, Kaniuk, Hillman, & Henderson, 2003). Beyond infancy, there is evidence of linear deterioration in the mental health of children entering foster care at progressively older ages, including increasing interpersonal behaviour problems suggestive of attachment disturbances (Tarren-Sweeney, 2008c). The attachment difficulties of late-placed children are more resistant to therapeutic change in response to markedly improved care. This is partly due to them having more 'established' internal representations of self and others. One study found that birth maternal representations of late-placed children are shaped by the extent of maltreatment in their mothers' care, which in turn influence both their representations of their foster mothers, and their mental health (Milan & Pinderhughes, 2000).

There is emerging evidence felt security is an important component of the psychosocial development and well-being of children and young people in care, and that their felt security is closely linked to perceived placement security. One study found that indicators of placement security independently predicted better mental health among pre-adolescent children in care (Tarren-Sweeney, 2008c), while another found that retrospectively measured 'felt security' was associated with positive outcomes for young adults after they left care (Cashmore & Paxman, 2006). Placement instability is a critical risk encountered more often by late-placed children (Tarren-Sweeney, 2008c). Placement breakdown most often occurs when caregivers are confronted by severely disruptive behaviour. But, placement instability accounts for further deterioration in children's mental health, over and above the difficulties children bring to their placements (Delfabbro & Barber, 2003; Newton, Litrownik, & Landsverk, 2000). This contributes to the spiralling decline in stability and functioning observed among children who endure repeated placement breakdowns. In many respects this pattern constitutes a 'developmental cascade' that involves both cumulative and progressive effects (Masten & Cicchetti, 2010), and which at a practical level becomes increasingly more difficult to reverse as successive placement breakdowns occur.

Taken together, these various research findings: support policies that promote permanency for children in long-term care; suggest that the therapeutic potential of foster and kinship care is greater for children placed at earlier ages (Tarren-Sweeney, 2008c); and conversely, that late placement of children with pre-existing attachment and mental health difficulties may have limited therapeutic potential (Delfabbro & Barber, 2003).

The neglect of children's mental health needs

The challenge of working with maltreated children before they enter care

"The endpoint of chronically experiencing catastrophic states of relational trauma in early life is a progressive impairment of the ability to adjust, take defensive action, or act on one's own behalf, and a blocking of the capacity to register affect and pain, all critical to survival."

(Schore, 2010: p.39)

"Interpersonal violence, especially violence experienced by children, is the largest single preventable cause of mental illness. What cigarette smoking is to the rest of medicine, early childhood violence is to psychiatry."

(Scharfstein, 2006)

Many children who enter the care system have lived with fear and with parents, carers and siblings who are frightened and/or frightening. As practitioners, we need to engage more fully both with the effects of exposure to violence on children's development, and with the longer-term consequences, such as children's violent behaviour to themselves and others as they grow up. Collectively, we have good understandings of what promotes and supports resilient responding in children and families, and similarly what predisposes children and parents to traumatic responding. We know how to intervene to help prevent future recurrences of violence in families, and we know how to help prevent violence.

The effects on children's development of exposure to fear and chronic emotional over arousal are well documented to include: somatic symptoms, lack of interest in activities, constantly moving and highly distractible, numbing and an inability to comfort self, repetitive play, the development of new fears, sleep difficulties and behaviour changes. A social learning perspective suggests that children are at risk of learning aggressive styles of conduct, reduced restraint and increased arousal to aggressive situations, of becoming desensitised to violence, with distorted views of conflict resolution (Browne & Herbert, 1997).

The Children in Need Census in Cheshire, UK (2003) found that in 41% of all Social Services Department cases, domestic violence was a significant factor. The children were twice as likely to experience mental health difficulties themselves and to live in households where parents and carers had mental health problems. They were also five times more likely to live in households where psychoactive substances were misused. Such complexity in children's lives demands a thoughtful, co-ordinated systemic response from the many professional agencies involved with these children and their families.

Myers et al. (2002) identify five forms of child abuse, which often co-occur: physical abuse; sexual abuse; emotional or psychological abuse; neglect, including failure to protect a child from danger; and exposure to violence between parents or carers, which includes both witnessing actual violence and living in a home where violence takes place. In the UK, the law relating to child protection was altered in 2005 to include witnessing domestic violence as a risk factor. The change in legislation came about in part, as a result of the research findings that the adverse effects on children's development of exposure to family violence were much the same as when they actually experienced physical violence.

In our therapeutic work with both victims and perpetrators of violence in the family, we put safety first (Cooper & Vetere, 2005). Not surprisingly, many family members we work with, do not have a sense of entitlement to their own safety, and as parents, are not well placed to teach their children how to keep themselves safe. So acts of omission are as important to consider as acts of commission, when helping family members take responsibility for their behaviour, stop the violence and prevent the intergenerational transmission of attitudes and practices that normalise and justify violent acts.

The challenge of working with maltreated children after they are placed in care or adoption

In these days of swingeing economic cuts in UK public sector services, it is difficult to argue for more resources. But those of us who work in the UK can consider how we use our existing resources to the benefit of these children. More social care and mental health care practitioners are undertaking systemic training, so they can work with complexity, practise integrative formulation of problems, and approach communication and role difficulties within the professional network. Increasingly, Child and Adolescent Mental Health Services in the UK, with the help of Next Generation care, are developing specialist pathways to provide services for looked after children. Similarly, the recent Munro Report, reviewing social work services after the death of baby P, has recommended that social workers reclaim their previous therapeutic role, lost from their curriculum in the 1990s when all psychiatric social workers were recalled into child protection teams for the sole function of assessment.

The major models of psychotherapy are concerned with promoting reflexivity and affect regulation. They are designed to help people manage emotional over-arousal and under-arousal, and to develop reflective and empathic capacity. There is a good evidence base for individual, group, couple and family work where violence is the concern, provided there is a clear safety methodology (Jory, Anderson, & Greer, 1997; Stith, Rosen, & McCollum, 2002). Much of the work involves identifying patterns of behaviour and conflict that escalate into violence, and helping people de-escalate these unhelpful patterns and to develop more constructive ways of coping. Very often, the triggers for escalation into violence are attachment based, that is, fears of rejection and abandonment, and oversensitivity to shame and shaming based in earlier experiences of humiliation, that lead to the experience of physiological flooding. This work explores two powerful interfaces: between earlier trauma responses and current violence, and between power and control, and love and affection. Thus it is essential to consider the intergenerational context of relational trauma, the meaning of violence and safety, learning and development, and behavioural scripts across the lifespan when doing both preventative work, and assessments for risk and safety.

Children adopted and fostered from the care system may be experiencing overt or masked trauma symptoms, such as nightmares, hyper-arousal, difficulties with concentration, behavioural problems, and so on. Despite trauma training and support for foster carers and adoptive parents, it is not always easy to make the link between relational/developmental trauma and the child's behaviour. As an example, a couple in their late 30s with no birth children of their own, had adopted a boy of 6. They had been living together for 6 months and the parents had approached the adoption agency, saying they could no longer live with the boy and look after him. On the suggestion of the agency, they attended a post-adoption consultation service, where they were seen by one of us (Arlene) and my colleague in a last ditch attempt to keep the boy living at home with them. The boy had been emotionally and physically neglected for the first 4 years of his life. In particular he had been denied food on a regular basis. The adoptive parents had attended all the adoption preparation workshops, including the ones on trauma responses in children. In talking with the parents, we learned about their distress and beliefs about the boy and his 'difficult' behaviour, and why they thought the adoption could not work. We asked for examples, and they told us the following story. The mother would cook a hot dinner for the evening meal. The boy would come into the kitchen 5 minutes before it was ready, whilst she prepared to dish up. He would demand food now. The mother would tell him dinner was nearly ready and show him through the glass in the oven door, the lasagne bubbling away nicely in the oven. She would tell him to wait a few minutes while she dished up. He would scream and demand food, and fling himself around the kitchen floor (zero to sixty in one second, as she put it). Such behaviour in the kitchen with a hot stove was dangerous and the father would come in to help. He would tell the boy off, and put him in his bedroom until he calmed down, thus delaying the boy's dinner time. The father was acting from an intergenerational script drawn from his own experience of being parented – the need to follow rules, do as you are told, and going to your bedroom to calm down. As we talked through this example with the adoptive parents, we reflected on the impact on a child of being denied food, and how in your new home, you may need to test the boundary of whether food would be given to you, or denied. We reflected on the relational trauma experienced by the boy and how this would show in a lack of trust. In this example, the parents decided to make food freely (and healthily!) available to the child, by putting small snack pots in the refrigerator that he could access at any time. They dropped their rule of not eating before dinner. Thus what had been seen as the boy's naughty behaviour had been reframed as an understandable response to having been denied food, in the context of trauma responding. The adoptive parents decided to continue with looking after the boy, and they accepted support from the consultation service, and with time, patience and a different set of understandings they grew to love and care for each other. The link between theory and practice and between theory and behaviour sometimes needs special and specialist support as trauma responses play out in people's lives in potentially disruptive and unregulated ways.

The mental health of children in care and those adopted from care

Surveys have consistently found that a child in care is more likely than not to have psychological difficulties of sufficient scale or severity to require mental health services, regardless of which country they reside in (Tarren-Sweeney, 2008a). Children in care also endure poorer physical health, higher prevalence of learning and language difficulties, and poorer educational outcomes than other children (Crawford, 2006). More than 20 population studies in North America, Europe and Australia have measured the mental health of children in care using standard caregiver-report rating scales – primarily the Child Behavior Checklist (CBCL) (Achenbach & Rescorla, 2001), the Strengths and Difficulties Questionnaire (SDQ) (Goodman, 2001) and the Rutter Scales (Elander & Rutter, 1996). These studies have consistently found that the scale of their mental health difficulties more closely resembles that of clinic-referred children, than of children at large (Armsden, Pecora, Payne, & Szatkiewicz, 2000; Burns et al., 2004; Cappelletty, Brown, & Shumate, 2005; Heflinger, Simpkins, & Combs-Orme, 2000; Pilowsky, 1995; Tarren-Sweeney & Hazell, 2006). Around half of children in care score in the clinical range on one or more CBCL broadband or syndrome scales, while around three-quarters score above one or more borderline range cut-points. Studies have also estimated high prevalence of DSM-III-R and DSM-IV Conduct Disorder (17%–45%), Attention-deficit Hyperactivity Disorder (10%–30%), Depression (4%–36%), Post-traumatic Stress Disorder (40%–50%), and Generalised Anxiety (or DSM-III-R Overanxious) Disorder (4%–26%) among mixed samples of children and young people in foster and residential care (Blower, Addo, Hodgson, Lamington, & Towlson, 2004; Dubner & Motta, 1999; Famularo & Augustyn, 1996; McCann, Wilson, & Dunn, 1996; McMillen, et al., 2005; Stein, Rae-Grant, Ackland, & Avison, 1994).

Children in residential care have greater mental health problems than those in family-type foster care (Hukkanen, Sourander, Bergroth, & Piha, 1999) while those in kinship care have less problems (Holtan, Ronning, Handegard, & Sourander, 2005). The extent to which these differences are attributable to different care experiences, versus selection, is unclear. Older age is associated with poorer mental health among children in care, as indicated by differences in age-standardised CBCL scores (Armsden, et al., 2000; Dubowitz, Zuravin, Starr, Feigelman, & Harrington, 1993; Heflinger, et al., 2000), but this age effect is confounded by *age at entry into care* (older children are more likely to have entered care at an older age and with poorer pre-care mental health) (Tarren-Sweeney, 2008c). There are inconsistent data regarding gender differences in mental health.

There has been little specific research on the mental health difficulties of children adopted from care. An eight-year longitudinal study of a small (n = 16) sample of primary school-aged boys adopted from foster care, found they had less conduct and emotional problems over time, whereas their overactivity and relationship difficulties persisted (Rushton, Treseder, & Quinton, 1995). Although children adopted from care enjoy greater placement stability than those who remain in care, studies carried out in England suggest as many as 60% of children manifest mental health difficulties six years after being adopted from care (Rushton, 2004; Selwyn, Sturgess, Quinton, & Baxter, 2006). A population survey presently being carried out by researchers at Great Ormond St Hospital London, has been designed to reveal a more complete picture of the mental health of children following adoption from care (personal communication, Margaret DeJong and Jill Hodges).

Characteristic difficulties that are not measured by standard survey instruments

Children and young people in care manifest a range of attachment- and trauma-related mental health difficulties that are under-researched, and inadequately measured by standard mental health measures, such as the CBCL and SDQ. The Assessment Checklist for Children (ACC) is a caregiver-report psychiatric rating scale that was developed to measure these difficulties in the longitudinal Children in Care Study (CICS, n = 347), carried out in New South Wales, Australia (Tarren-Sweeney, 2007). Findings from the CICS baseline survey suggest that around half of children in care manifest one or more forms of clinically meaningful attachment-related interpersonal behaviour difficulties, and sizeable proportions display clinically significant self-injury (7%) and abnormal responses to pain (5%) (Tarren-Sweeney & Hazell, 2006). A pattern of excessive eating and food maintenance behaviour without concurrent obesity was also identified, resembling the behavioural correlates of Hyperphagic Short Stature (Psychosocial Dwarfism) (Tarren-Sweeney, 2006). Up to a third of children presented with problematic sexual behaviour, which for some is possibly mediated by attachment difficulties (Friedrich, et al., 2005; Tarren-Sweeney, 2008b).

Patterns and complexity of mental health difficulties

More is known about the scale and prevalence of mental health difficulties experienced by children and young people in out-of-home care, than of their nature, patterns or complexity. This is largely because most available data were obtained as outcome measures in studies addressing non-clinical research questions. However, recent findings suggest that a sizeable proportion manifest complex psychopathology, characterised by attachment difficulties, relationship insecurity, problematic sexual behaviour, trauma-related anxiety, inattention/hyperactivity, and conduct problems and defiance (Tarren-Sweeney, 2008a).

A series of cluster analyses performed on CBCL and ACC scores obtained in the CICS survey identified several complex symptom clusters (Tarren-Sweeney, In Press). Among the CICS sample:

- Thirty per cent of children were reported with normative difficulties
- Fifteen per cent had elevated, sub-clinical checklist scores
- Thirty-five per cent had relatively non-complex, clinically significant psychopathology (that could reasonably be conceptualised as discrete mental disorders or co-morbidity within standard diagnostic classifications)
- Twenty per cent manifested *complex attachment- and trauma-related psychopathology that is not adequately conceptualised within standard classification.*

The CICS analyses indicate that the presence of hallmark social and interpersonal relationship difficulties among a large proportion of children in care – which overlays and possibly mediates children's experience of other types of symptoms – adds to symptom complexity. This complexity accounts for some surprising results. For example, despite a high prevalence of clinical-level DSM-oriented attention-deficit hyperactivity scores among the CICS sample (Tarren-Sweeney & Hazell, 2006), an ADHD profile type was not located for either gender. Instead, various analyses suggest that clinically significant inattention/over-activity among children in the CICS was largely manifested as a component of complex symptomatology.

There were some distinct differences between the derived symptom profiles that merit further research, and which suggest new ways of conceptualising complex attachment- and trauma-related disorders. Beyond this, however, the profiles *do not* provide a basis for a taxonomy of complex attachment- and trauma-related disorders. The clusters were differentiated more by profile elevation than profile shape or pattern, suggesting an absence of *typology*. Furthermore, whilst the cluster analyses yielded statistically delineated symptom profile types, their clinical distinctness is questionable. Close inspection of children's individual score profiles showed a lack of clear delineation between the derived profile types, and considerable variability between children's symptom profiles. This implies that any taxonomy of complex attachment- and trauma-related disorders is likely to have poor specificity. It may be that much of the symptomatology identified in the CICS is both too complex, and shows too much variability across children's individual profiles, to allow for traditional classification.

What do we know about their use of mental health services?

The availability of mental health services for children and young people in care (and for those subsequently adopted), and the extent to which adults and agencies responsible for their well-being act to obtain such services, is a critical public health and humanitarian concern. As described earlier in this chapter, studies have consistently established that more than half of children in care, regardless of where they reside in the western world, have mental health problems of sufficient scale and severity to warrant the provision of mental health services. Indeed, it can be argued that no other non-clinically defined child population has greater need for mental health services.

In spite of this apparent need, various studies have suggested that sizeable proportions of children and young people in care who might benefit from intervention, do not receive adequate clinical assessment or access to mental health services – either because:

- Their difficulties remain undetected
- Services are not sought by their social workers or caregivers
- They are unable to access available services
- There is a lack of suitable services.

(Kerker & Dore, 2006; Minnis, Everett, Pelosi, Dunn, & Knapp, 2006; Sawyer, Carbone, Searle, & Robinson, 2007)

This is despite governments holding parental responsibility obligations for these children. While it is reported that maltreated US children are more likely to access public mental health services following entry into care than when they were in their parents' care (Leslie et al., 2005), rates of service use fall well short of the estimated rate requiring mental health services. Low rates of service use have also been found among children in care in Scotland (Minnis et al., 2006) and South Australia (Sawyer et al., 2007). An exception was found in the aforementioned CICS survey in NSW, Australia, where around three-quarters of children with clinically meaningful mental health difficulties were receiving mental health services (Tarren-Sweeney, 2010).

Among children and young people adopted from care, there is evidence that (in the UK at least) their access to mental health services increases after they are adopted. In one study, whereas 26% of children adopted from care had accessed CAMHS prior to their adoption (Sturgess & Selwyn, 2007), this rate increased to more than 55% following adoption – which exceeds the rate of mental health service use among all children in the CICS sample (Tarren-Sweeney, 2010).

A low level of unmet demand for mental health services was found in the CICS survey, with only 12% of caregivers saying they had been unsuccessful in accessing mental health services. While this was an unexpected finding, it can be partially explained by the provision of a Psychology service within the state child welfare department in NSW, Australia. Access to generic

CAMHS and other clinical services in NSW was also possibly facilitated through the introduction of 'best endeavours' legislation, which effectively prioritises access to human services by child welfare clients in that state. The situation in NSW then is probably more favourable than in most other jurisdictions in the western world. Despite this, caregivers neither accessed nor sought mental health services for around a quarter of children with clinically significant mental health difficulties, reinforcing previous findings that foster caregivers represent a critical gateway to mental health services (Tarren-Sweeney, 2010).

Correlates and predictors of mental health service use

A number of (mostly US) studies have attempted to locate pathways and barriers to clinical services by identifying the correlates and predictors of service delivery. This includes prospective data for a large, nationally representative sample of child welfare clients (including children in care), obtained in the National Survey of Child and Adolescent Well-being (NSCAW) (NSCAW Research Group, 2002). A moderate correlation between children's symptom scores on standardised checklists, and their use of mental health services has been found in studies in the US and Australia (Bellamy, 2007; Burns et al., 2004; Garland, Landsverk, Hough, & Ellis-Macleod, 1996; Leslie, et al., 2000; Tarren-Sweeney, 2010; Zima, Bussing, Yang, & Belin, 2000), while in the aforementioned Scottish survey, children's access and/or use of mental health services was found to be unrelated to the number and severity of their mental health symptoms (Minnis et al., 2006).

The relationships between children's use of mental health services and the *types of difficulties* they manifest are less clear. In the CICS, mental health service use was unrelated to broad typology of DSM-IV disorders (i.e. internalising versus externalising versus ADHD disorders) (Tarren-Sweeney, 2010). Instead, it was found that children with greater symptom complexity and severity were more likely to obtain services, as indicated by clinical scores across two or more of the three typologies. This contrasts with findings elsewhere that children in care who have attention-deficit/hyperactivity symptoms are more likely to receive services than those with other symptoms or disorders (Minnis et al., 2006; Zima et al., 2000); and that foster youth with conduct problems have greater difficulty accessing services, in some cases due to active exclusion of children with disruptive behaviours (Kerker & Dore, 2006).

The relationship between children's ethnicity or minority status and their access to mental health services whilst in care, is likely to vary across the western world. In the United States, while African-American children in care may show a better match between symptom severity and use of services as compared to equivalent Caucasian children (Garland et al., 2000), they also have considerably less access to mental health services overall (Bellamy, 2007; Leslie, Hurlburt, Landsverk, Barth, & Slymen, 2004; Zima et al.,

2000). Another demographic predictor of access to mental health services for this population is older age (Bellamy, 2007) which may serve as a marker for higher rates of disruptive behaviour. The relationship between gender and children's access to mental health services remains unclear because of conflicting and inconclusive findings (Bellamy, 2007; Blumberg, Landsverk, Ellis-MacLeod, Ganger, & et al., 1996; Burns, et al., 2004; Tarren-Sweeney, 2010).

Several studies have found that active forms of maltreatment (most notably sexual abuse), predict higher use of mental health services, after controlling for the scale of their mental health symptoms – whereas children who only experience neglect are much less likely to receive services (Bellamy, 2007; Garland et al., 1996; Leslie et al., 2004). However, it is questionable whether one can make valid distinctions between active forms of abuse and neglect among children with a background of severe, complex and chronic maltreatment.

Finally, it is likely that the heterogeneity of social care and public health systems throughout the western world accounts for considerable variation in mental health service *access* and *use* by children and young people in care, and those who are subsequently adopted. We believe the findings described in this section do not offer clear guidance to policy makers outside of the US, NSW and perhaps Scotland. We therefore believe that policy makers in other locations should obtain *local* data on access to mental health services by children in care in their country, province or region – particularly when planning for specialised service delivery.

References

Achenbach, T., & Rescorla, L. (2001). *Manual for ASEBA school-age forms and profiles*. Burlington, VT: University of Vermont, Research Center for Children, Youth, & Families.

Armsden, G., Pecora, P. J., Payne, V. H., & Szatkiewicz, J. P. (2000). 'Children placed in long-term foster care: An intake profile using the child behavior checklist/4-18'. *Journal of Emotional & Behavioral Disorders*, 8(1), 49–64.

Australian Institute of Health and Welfare. (2012). *Child protection Australia 2010 – 2011*. Child Welfare Series no. 53. Canberra: AIHW.

Bellamy, J. (2007). *Mental health need, outpatient service use, and outcomes among children who have experienced long-term foster care*. Unpublished Dissertation, Columbia University, New York.

Biehal, N., Ellison, S., Baker, C., & Sinclair, I. (2009). *Characteristics, outcomes and meanings of three types of permanent placement: Adoption by strangers, adoption by carers, and long-term foster care*. London: Department for Children Schools and Families (DCSF).

Blower, A., Addo, A., Hodgson, J., Lamington, L., & Towlson, K. (2004). 'Mental Health of "Looked after" Children: A Needs Assessment'. *Clinical Child Psychology and Psychiatry*, 9, 117–129.

Blumberg, E., Landsverk, J., Ellis-MacLeod, E., Ganger, W., Culver, S. (1996). 'Use of the public mental health system by children in foster care: Client characteristics and service use patterns'. *Journal of Mental Health Administration*, 23(4), 389–405.

Bowlby, J. (1988). *A secure base: Clinical applications of attachment theory*. London: Routledge.
Browne, K., & Herbert, M. (1997). *Preventing family violence*. Chichester: Wiley.
Burns, B. J., Phillips, S., Wagner, H., Barth, R. P., Kolko, D., Campbell, Y., et al. (2004). 'Mental health need and access to mental health services by youths involved with child welfare: A national survey'. *Journal of the American Academy of Child & Adolescent Psychiatry*, 43(8), 960–970.
Cappelletty, G., Brown, M., & Shumate, S. (2005). 'Correlates of the Randolph Attachment Disorder Questionnaire (RADQ) in a sample of children in foster placement'. *Child and Adolescent Social Work Journal*, 22(1), 71–84.
Cashmore, J., & Paxman, M. (2006). 'Predicting after-care outcomes: The importance of "felt" security'. *Child and Family Social Work*, 11, 232–241.
Cicchetti, D., Toth, S. L., & Maughan, A. (2000). 'An ecological-transactional model of child maltreatment'. In A. Sameroff & M. Lewis (Eds.), *Handbook of developmental psychopathology (2nd ed.)* (pp. 689-722). Dordrecht, Netherlands: Kluwer Academic Publishers.
Cooper, J., & Vetere, A. (2005). *Domestic violence and family safety: A systemic approach to working with violence in families*. Chichester: Wiley.
Crawford, M. (2006). 'Health of children in out-of-home care: Can we do better?'. *Journal of Paediatrics & Child Health*, 42, 77–78.
Crittenden, P. M., & Ainsworth, M. D. S. (1989). 'Child maltreatment and attachment theory'. In D. Cicchetti & V. Carlson (Eds.), *Child maltreatment: Theory and research on the causes and consequences of child abuse and neglect* (pp. 432–463). New York, NY: Cambridge University Press.
Delfabbro, P. H., & Barber, J. G. (2003). 'Before it's too late: Enhancing the early detection and prevention of long-term placement disruption'. *Children Australia*, 28(2), 14–18.
Department for Education. (2011). *Children looked after in England (including adoption and care leavers) year ending 31 March 2011*. London: Department for Education.
Dozier, M., Stovall, K. C., Albus, K. E., & Bates, B. (2001). 'Attachment for infants in foster care: The role of caregiver state of mind'. *Child Development*, 72(5), 1467–1477.
Dubner, A. E., & Motta, R. W. (1999). 'Sexually and physically abused foster care children and post traumatic stress disorder'. *Journal of Consulting and Clinical Psychology*, 67(3), 367–373.
Dubowitz, H., Zuravin, S., Starr, R. H., Feigelman, S., & Harrington, D. (1993). 'Behavior problems of children in kinship care'. *Journal of Developmental and Behavioral Pediatrics*, 14(6), 386–393.
Elander, J., & Rutter, M. (1996). 'Use and development of the Rutter parents' and teachers' scales'. *International Journal of Methods in Psychiatric Research*, 6(2), 63–78.
Famularo, R., & Augustyn, M. (1996). 'Persistence of pediatric post traumatic stress disorder after 2 years'. *Child Abuse and Neglect*, 20(12).
Fanshel, D., & Shinn, E. (1978). *Children in foster care: A longitudinal investigation*. New York: Columbia University Press.
Fergusson, D., & Lynskey, M. (1996). 'Adolescent resiliency to family adversity'. *Journal of Child Psychology & Psychiatry*, 33, 1059–1075.
Friedrich, W. N., Baker, A., Parker, R., Schneiderman, M., Gries, L., & Archer, M. (2005). 'Youth with problematic sexualised behaviors in the child welfare system: A one-year longitudinal study'. *Sexual Abuse*, 17(4), 391–406.

Garland, A. F., Hough, R. L., Landsverk, J. A., McCabe, K. M., Yeh, M., Ganger, W. C., et al. (2000). 'Racial and ethnic variations in mental health care utilization among children in foster care'. *Children's Services: Social Policy, Research, and Practice*, 3(3), 133–146.

Garland, A. F., Landsverk, J. L., Hough, R. L., & Ellis-Macleod, E. (1996). 'Type of maltreatment as a predictor of mental health service use for children in foster care'. *Child Abuse & Neglect*, 20(8), 675–688.

Goodman, R. (2001). 'Psychometric properties of the Strengths and Difficulties Questionnaire'. *Journal of the American Academy of Child & Adolescent Psychiatry*, 40, 1337–1345.

Heflinger, C. A., Simpkins, C. G., & Combs-Orme, T. (2000). 'Using the CBCL to determine the clinical status of children in state custody'. *Children & Youth Services Review*, 22(1), 55–73.

Holtan, A., Ronning, J., Handegard, B., & Sourander, A. (2005). 'A comparison of mental health problems in kinship and nonkinship foster care'. *European Child and Adolescent Psychiatry*, 14(4), 200–207.

Holzer, P., & Bromfield, L. (2008). *NCPASS comparability of child protection data: Project report*. Melbourne: Australian Institute of Family Studies.

Howe, D., & Fearnley, S. (2003). 'Disorders of Attachment in Adopted and Fostered Children: Recognition and Treatment'. *Clinical Child Psychology & Psychiatry*, 8, 369–387.

Hukkanen, R., Sourander, A., Bergroth, L., & Piha, J. (1999). 'Psychosocial factors and adequacy of services for children in children's homes'. *European Child and Adolescent Psychiatry*, 8, 268–275.

Johnson, R. L., Browne, K., & Hamilton-Giachritsis, C. (2006). 'Young children in institutional care at risk of harm'. *Trauma, Violence and Abuse* 7(1), 34–60.

Kerker, B., & Dore, M. (2006). 'Mental health needs and treatment of foster youth: Barriers and opportunities'. *American Journal of Orthopsychiatry*, 76(1), 138–147.

Leslie, L., Hurlburt, M., James, S., Landsverk, J., Slymen, D. J., & Zhang, J. (2005). 'Relationship between entry into child welfare and mental health service use'. *Psychiatric Services*, 56(8), 981–987.

Leslie, L., Hurlburt, M., Landsverk, J., Barth, R. P., & Slymen, D. J. (2004). 'Outpatient mental health services for children in foster care: A national perspective'. *Child Abuse & Neglect*, 28, 697–712.

Leslie, L., Landsverk, J., Ezzet-Lofstrom, R., Tschann, J. M., Slymen, D. J., & Garland, A. F. (2000). 'Children in foster care: Factors influencing outpatient mental health service use'. *Child Abuse & Neglect*, 24(4), 465–476.

Lock, J. A. (1997). *The Aboriginal child placement principle: research project no. 7*. Sydney: New South Wales Law Reform Commission.

Marcus, R. F. (1991). 'The attachments of children in foster care'. *Genetic, Social, & General Psychology Monographs*, 117(4), 365–394.

Masten, A. S., & Cicchetti, D. (2010). 'Editorial: Developmental cascades'. *Development and Psychopathology*, 22, 491–495.

McCann, J., Wilson, S., & Dunn, G. (1996). 'Prevalence of psychiatric disorders in young people in the care system'. *British Medical Journal*, 313, 1529–1530.

McMillen, J. C., Zima, B. T., Scott, L., Auslander, W., Munson, M., Ollie, M., et al. (2005). 'Prevalence of psychiatric disorders among older youths in the foster care system'. *Journal of the American Academy of Child & Adolescent Psychiatry*, 44(1), 88–95.

Milan, S. E., & Pinderhughes, E. E. (2000). 'Factors influencing maltreated children's early adjustment in foster care'. *Development and Psychopathology*, 12(1), 63–81.

Minnis, H., Everett, K., Pelosi, A., Dunn, J., & Knapp, M. (2006). 'Children in foster care: Mental health, service use and costs'. *European Child and Adolescent Psychiatry*, 15, 63–70.

Myers, J., Berliner, L., Briere, J., Hendrix, C., Jenny, C., & Reid, T. (2002). *The APSAC handbook on child maltreatment* (2nd ed.). Thousand Oaks, CA: Sage.

Newman, L., & Mares, S. (2007). 'Recent advances in the theories of and interventions with attachment disorders'. *Current Opinion in Psychiatry*, 20, 343–348.

Newton, R. R., Litrownik, A. J., & Landsverk, J. A. (2000). 'Children and youth in foster care: Disentangling the relationship between problem behaviors and number of placements'. *Child Abuse and Neglect*, 24(10), 1363–1374.

NSCAW Research Group. (2002). 'Methodological lessons from the National Survey of Child and Adolescent Well-being: The first three years of the USA's first national probability study of children and families investigated for abuse and neglect'. *Children & Youth Services Review*, 24(6/7), 513–541.

Nutt, L. (2006). *The lives of foster carers: Private sacrifices, public restrictions*. Abingdon Oxon: Routledge.

O'Connor, T., Bredenkamp, D., Rutter, M., & the English and Romanian Adoptees Study Team. (1999). 'Attachment disturbances and disorders in children exposed to early severe deprivation'. *Infant Mental Health Journal*, 20(1), 10–29.

O'Connor, T., & Zeanah, C. (2003). 'Attachment disorders: Assessment strategies and treatment approaches'. *Attachment and Human Development*, 5(3), 223–244.

Pilowsky, D. (1995). 'Psychopathology among children placed in family foster care'. *Psychiatric Services*, 46(9), 906–910.

Plomin, R., DeFries, J., & McClearn, G. (1997). *Behavioral genetics* (3rd ed.). New York: W.H. Freeman.

Rushton, A. (2004). 'A scoping and scanning review of research on the adoption of children placed from foster care'. *Clinical Child Psychology & Psychiatry*, 9(1), 89–106.

Rushton, A., Treseder, J., & Quinton, D. (1995). 'An eight-year prospective study of older boys placed in permanent substitute families: A research note'. *Journal of Child Psychology & Psychiatry & Allied Disciplines*, 36(4), 687–695.

Rutter, M. (1999). 'Psychosocial adversity and child psychopathology'. *British Journal of Psychiatry*, 174, 480–493.

——(2000). 'Children in substitute care: Some conceptual considerations and research implications'. *Children & Youth Services Review*, 22(9-10), 685–703.

Sawyer, M. G., Carbone, J. A., Searle, A. K., & Robinson, P. (2007). 'The mental health and well-being of children and adolescents in home-based foster care'. *Medical Journal of Australia*, 186, 181–184.

Scharfstein, S. (2006). *Task force on the effects of violence on children*. Washington, DC: American Psychiatric Association.

Schofield, G. (2002). 'The significance of a secure base: A psychosocial model of long-term foster care'. *Child & Family Social Work*, 7, 259–272.

Schofield, G., & Ward, E. (2008). *Permanence in foster care: a study of care planning and practice in England and Wales*. London: BAAF.

Schore, A. (2010). 'Relational trauma and the developing right brain: The neurobiology of broken attachment bonds'. In T. Brandon (Ed.), *Relational trauma in infancy*. London: Routledge.

Selwyn, J., Sturgess, W., Quinton, D., & Baxter, C. (2006). *Costs and outcomes of non-infant adoptions*. London: BAAF.
Steele, M., Hodges, J., Kaniuk, J., Hillman, S., & Henderson, K. (2003). 'Attachment representations and adoption: Associations between maternal states of mind and emotion narratives in previously maltreated children'. *Journal of Child Psychotherapy, 29*(2), 187–205.
Stein, E., Rae-Grant, N., Ackland, S., & Avison, W. (1994). 'Psychiatric disorders of children "in care": Methodology and demographic correlates'. *Canadian Journal of Psychiatry. Revue Canadienne de Psychiatrie, 39*(6), 341–347.
Sturgess, W., & Selwyn, J. (2007). 'Supporting the placements of children adopted out of care'. *Clinical Child Psychology and Psychiatry, 12*(1), 13–28.
Tarren-Sweeney, M. (2006). 'Patterns of aberrant eating among pre-adolescent children in foster care'. *Journal of Abnormal Child Psychology, 34*, 623–634.
——(2007). 'The Assessment Checklist for Children - ACC: A behavioral rating scale for children in foster, kinship and residential care'. *Children & Youth Services Review, 29*, 672–691.
——(2008a). 'The mental health of children in out-of-home care'. *Current Opinion in Psychiatry, 21*, 345–349.
——(2008b). 'Predictors of problematic sexual behavior among children with complex maltreatment histories'. *Child Maltreatment, 13*(2), 182–198.
——(2008c). 'Retrospective and concurrent predictors of the mental health of children in care'. *Children & Youth Services Review, 30*, 1–25.
——(2010). 'Concordance of mental health impairment and service utilisation among children in care'. *Clinical Child Psychology and Psychiatry, 15*(4), 481–495.
——(In Press). 'An investigation of complex attachment- and trauma-related symptomatology among children in foster and kinship care'. *Child Psychiatry and Human Development*. Online first, DOI: 10.1007/s10578-013-0366-x.
Tarren-Sweeney, M., & Hazell, P. (2006). 'The mental health of children in foster and kinship care in New South Wales, Australia'. *Journal of Paediatrics & Child Health, 42*, 91–99.
Zeanah, C., Boris, N. W., & Larrieu, J. A. (1997). 'Infant development and developmental risk: A review of the past 10 years'. *Journal of the American Academy of Child & Adolescent Psychiatry, 36*(2), 165–178.
Zima, B. T., Bussing, R., Yang, X., & Belin, T. R. (2000). 'Help-seeking steps and service use for children in foster care.' *Journal of Behavioral Health Services & Research, 27*(3), 271–228.

2 The benefits of outpatient mental health services for children in long-term foster care[1]

Jennifer Bellamy, Geetha Gopalan and Dorian Traube

Summary

Despite the tremendous mental health need evidenced by children in foster care and their high rates of use of mental health services, little is known about the impact of outpatient mental health services on the behavioral health of this population. This chapter describes a study which utilized data from the National Survey of Child and Adolescent Well-being (NSCAW), the first nationally representative study of child welfare in the United States. A sub-sample of 439 children who have experienced long-term foster care were included in this study. These data were used to estimate the impact of outpatient mental health services on the externalizing and internalizing behavior problems of children in long-term foster care. A propensity score matching model was employed to produce a robust estimate of the treatment effect. Results indicate that children who have experienced long-term foster care do not benefit from the receipt of outpatient mental health services. Study results are discussed in the context of earlier research on the quality of mental health services for children in foster care.

Introduction

This chapter describes a study of the effectiveness of outpatient mental health services for children in foster care, using data from the National Survey of Child and Adolescent Well-being (NSCAW) – the first nationally representative study of child welfare in the United States. Children in foster care manifest notably higher rates of behavioral problems (Burns et al., 2004) and greater use of mental health services as compared to youth in the general population (Becker, Jordan, & Larsen, 2006; Landsverk, Slymen & Leslie, 2004; Leslie, Hurlburt, Landsverk, Barth, & Slymen, 2004; Leslie et al., 2005). However, little is known about the actual impact of mental health service provision for the population of children in out-of-home care. As multiple factors other than mental health treatment have been linked to the behavioral health of children in foster care, measuring the unique impact of mental health services can be challenging. Consequently, we carried out a study designed to isolate the impact of outpatient mental health services from these factors and offer an estimate of the effect of providing outpatient mental health services to children in foster care. In this chapter we use the terms foster care and out-of-home care interchangeably.

Mental health needs and service utilisation of children in foster care

As many as 80% of youth in the United States with active child welfare cases present with behavioral or emotional disorders, developmental delays, and other health and mental health problems (Leslie et al., 2005a). Nationally representative studies have identified that 47.9% of child welfare involved youth score in the clinical range on the Child Behavior Check List (CBCL) (Achenbach, 1991; Burns, et al., 2004). Maltreated youth involved in the child welfare system are 2.5 times more likely to have a mental health need as compared to children in the general population (Burns et al., 2004).

The rate of service use for this population further underscores their high level of need. Children in out-of-home foster care manifest greater levels of mental health service utilization as compared to children who live in poverty (Administration for Children and Families, 2005; Geen, Sommers, & Cohen, 2005; Leslie et al., 2005b; Stahmer et al., 2005). Moreover, children in foster care are more likely to receive mental health services than youth with child welfare contact who remain at home (Burns et al., 2004; Leslie et al., 2005). The child welfare system has been characterized as a gateway to mental health services (Stiffman, Pescosolido, & Cabassa, 2004) and entry into foster care appears to represent one of the largest keys to that gateway.

Despite the high need and the high rates of service use, little is actually known about the impact of these services on children's behavioral health outcomes. Studies of outpatient child mental health services in child welfare reveal that the intensity and quality of services provided to children in foster care varies widely (McKay et al., 2004). Unfortunately, '... there is little empirical basis for the notion that a higher frequency of services invariably translates into improved outcome' (James et al., 2004, p. 137). Coordination of care studies suggests that increased use of formal child mental health treatment does not translate into fewer behavioral or emotional difficulties (Bickman, Smith, Lambert, & Andrade, 2003).

Furthermore, formal mental health services may not always be needed for children in foster care in spite of high rates of clinical need. For instance, many children with substantial mental health difficulties who do not receive services, both inside and outside of foster care, often improve without treatment (Burns et al. 2004; Lambert & Bickman, 2004).

Factors contributing to mental health difficulties and service use

A host of factors, including child maltreatment, sociodemographic characteristics, placement stability and placement type, have been frequently linked to both children's behavioral health and use of mental health services. We briefly explore each of these factors.

The experience of maltreatment can lead to a host of mental health concerns for youth (Cicchetti & Toth, 2004; Kaplow & Widom, 2007; Leslie, Gordon et al., 2005; Springer, Sheridan, Kuo, & Carnes, 2007), and maltreatment is sometimes conceptualized as an indicator of mental health service need in and of itself (McMillen et al., 2004). Not surprisingly, research has linked more severe abuse to greater levels of emotional and behavioral problems among children and well into adulthood (Bradley et al., 2011; Burns et al., 2004; Oshri, Rogosch, Burnette, & Cicchetti, 2011). Certain types of maltreatment, such as physical and sexual abuse, have also been associated with a greater mental health service use (Burns et al., 2004; Leslie et al., 2004), while other studies have found no relationship between maltreatment type and mental health service utilization (Tarren-Sweeney, 2010). Any association with maltreatment type and mental health service use may not reflect an actual increase in mental health need related to these forms of maltreatment (Lambert & Bickman, 2004). Rather, mental health service use may reflect the perception that certain forms of maltreatment, such as physical and sexual abuse, result in relatively more harm than other forms of maltreatment (Garland et al., 1996). If caseworkers and caregivers perceive certain forms of abuse to be more harmful by nature, then children who have a history may be more likely to be referred to mental health services regardless of measurable clinical need.

The sociodemographic characteristics associated with differences in mental health status among children involved in the child welfare system include gender, age, socio-economic status and race/ethnicity. For example, older children frequently display greater mental health need than young children (e.g. Administration for Children and Families, 2005; Burns et al., 2004; Leslie et al., 2004; Raghavan et al., 2005), while young children (ages 2–5 years old) are more likely to access mental health services than older children (Burns et al., 2004). Differences in lifetime prevalence of PTSD, substance abuse and depression have been found to vary by gender and race/ethnicity among adolescents in the child welfare system (Keller, Salazar, & Courtney, 2010). Background characteristics such as child gender, having a parent with a criminal history, and low income have been found to be stronger predictors of mental health need than entry into out-of-home care (Stein et al., 1996). Some of these sociodemographic characteristics have also been linked to access to care. For example, race/ethnic disparities in mental health services use among children involved in the child welfare system has been found in a number of studies (Burns et al., 2004).

Arguably two of the most important adults for children in foster care are foster caregivers and foster care caseworkers. Foster caregivers and caseworkers can, and do, intervene when children are struggling with behavioral problems (Buehler, Rhodes, Orme, & Cuddeback, 2006; Cox, Orme, & Rhodes, 2003; Leathers, et al., 2009). For example, if caseworkers accurately perceive that a child is in need of mental health services, that caseworker is more likely to serve as a gateway provider and facilitate mental health services for the child (Stiffman, Pescosolido, & Cabassa, 2004).

For children in out-of-home care, foster care placement stability has also been consistently associated with children's behavioral health. Children who have behavioral problems, particularly externalizing behaviour difficulties, are more likely to experience placement disruptions. Likewise, placement disruptions can also lead to increased emotional and behavioral symptoms (Aarons, James, Monn, Raghavan, Wells, & Leslie, 2010).

The type of out-of-home care a child experiences can also have an impact on both need for and use of mental health services. For example, children who are placed with kinship caregivers use fewer mental health services (James et al., 2004). However, it is difficult to say if this relationship between kin placement and relatively low service utilization is due to less need for mental health services, or differences in help-seeking by kin versus non-kin caregivers. Kin caregivers in the United States tend to be less educated (Cuddeback, 2004), and caregiver education is linked to increased service use (Kerker & Dore, 2006). Also, children in kin placements experience more stability and fewer placement changes. Given that placement disruption has been consistently linked to children's behavior problems (Aarons et al., 2010; Cuddeback, 2004), children in kinship care are likely to have less mental health need compared to children in non-kinship placements.

One challenge related to isolating the impact of outpatient mental health services for children who have experienced long-term foster care are the multitude of factors described above that can relate to both need for and access to service. The purpose of this chapter is to explicitly account for these important and confounding factors and produce an estimate of the effect of outpatient mental health services on the behavioral health of children in long-term foster care in the United States. To do so, we employ propensity score matching, an analogue to a randomised controlled trial using observational data, to estimate this effect.

The National Survey of Child and Adolescent Well-Being

Sample

Data for this study were drawn from the long-term foster care subsample of the National Survey of Child and Adolescent Well-Being (NSCAW). The NSCAW sample of children was selected using a two-stage combined stratification and cluster design. In the first stage, the US was divided into nine strata. The majority of children served by the US child welfare system reside in eight states, which constituted the first eight strata. The ninth and final stratum consisted of the remaining 42 states and the District of Columbia. Within each stratum individual areas served by a single Child Protective Service (CPS) agency constituted the primary sampling units (PSUs). The PSU sampling frame included all service areas with approximately 60 or more cases per year. The smaller service areas that were not included in the sampling frame constituted about 3% of all cases nationally. One hundred PSUs were randomly selected from each stratum using a probability-proportionate-to-size procedure. Of the 100 PSUs selected, eight were considered ineligible because they were in states requiring first contact with the target child's caregiver to be made by a CPS worker, rather than an NSCAW field representative.

The NSCAW data include a sub-sample of children who experienced long-term foster care. The primary study eligibility requirements for the long-term foster care sample were: (1) out-of-home care for approximately 12 months at the time of sampling, (2) placement into out-of-home care preceded by an investigation of child maltreatment or a period of in-home services, and (3) out-of-home care at the time the sampling frame was produced. Only one child per household was included in the frame for sample selection. Eligible children were randomly sampled from children placed into care between July 1998 and February 1999. Therefore, children in this study had been in care somewhere between 8 and 18 months at sampling. This final sample was weighted, and these weights reflect both the probability of the PSU and the child's selection. Data for this study included the first three waves of the study collected at baseline, as well as at the 9-month and 18-month follow-ups.

Not all of the 727 children in the long-term foster care sample of the NSCAW were included in our study. Children under the age of two were excluded from the sample because of the lack of an appropriate measure of behavior problems for very young children. Also dropped from analyses were children who were no longer in foster care at the time that the baseline data were collected. Among children in out-of-home care, those who are placed in group care or other residential treatment centers generally have the highest rates of behavior problems (Administration for Children and Families, 2005). Typically, these placements are highly structured in nature and often utilize a number of behavioral interventions within the care setting. Because of the unique nature of these placements that integrate mental health services, and the particularly high rate of need among these children, youth in group care were also excluded from our study.

Measures

Outcomes

The outcomes for this study included externalizing and internalizing behavior problems as measured using Achenbach's (1991) Child Behavior

Checklist (CBCL) at 18-month follow-up. The CBCL was completed by the child's current caregiver. The CBCL has been used frequently throughout research on similar populations in both foster care and mental health studies, with well-established reliability and validity (Strijker, Zandberg, & van der Meulen, 2005; Xinsheng, Kaiser, & Hancock, 2004). The standardized scores of the CBCL measured at baseline were also used to control for existing behavior problems.

Treatment

Use of mental health services was measured using an adapted version of the Child and Adolescent Services Assessment (CASA), which appears to have good concurrent validity for outpatient services (K = 0.81) when compared to administrative reports of service use (Ascher, Farmer, Burns, & Angold, 1996; Farmer, Angold, Burns, & Costello, 1994). The CASA captures service use across 31 settings, including outpatient mental health services. Outpatient mental health services included day or partial hospitalization, outpatient drug or alcohol clinics, mental health centers, community health centers, crisis centers, and private professional treatment. This study utilized caregiver reports of service use. Children whose caregivers reported three or more outpatient mental health service visits were considered to have used outpatient mental health services.

Covariates

Covariates measured at baseline and used in this study included: (1) baseline behavioral problems; (2) caseworker's perceived need for care; (3) sociodemographic characteristics; (4) foster caregiver's report of their educational level; (5) maltreatment harm/severity; (6) placement type (kin or non-kin care); (7) the number of days that the child had been living in his or her current placement as reported by the caregiver as a proxy for placement stability; and (8) type of maltreatment.

Children's sociodemographic variables for the analyses included the child's race/ethnicity, gender and age. These variables were derived from administrative data, caregiver, and child self-reports. As a proxy measure for poverty, this study utilized caregivers' reports of current household receipt of government assistance, including WIC (Women Infants and Children), TANF (Temporary Assistance for Needy Families), or food stamps.

Caseworkers reported the type of maltreatment experienced by the child using a modified version of the Maltreatment Classification Scale (Manly, Cicchetti, & Barnett, 1994). The most severe form of maltreatment reported was used in this study and collapsed into four categories: sexual abuse, physical abuse, neglect, and other forms of maltreatment. The caseworker's perception of the degree of harm experienced by the child as a result of maltreatment was employed as a measure of the severity of the children's maltreatment experience. Caseworkers responded to the following question, 'Regardless of the outcome of the investigation, how would you describe the level of harm to [the child]?' and rated the severity on a scale ranging from 1 'None' to 4 'Severe'.

Analyses

Analyses for the study were performed using Stata Statistical Software Release 10 (StataCorp, 2007). STATA's survey commands accounted for the NSCAW's sampling and weighting strategy. Multiple imputation (MI) was employed to address missing data. In simulation studies, MI generally outperforms other approaches, such as listwise deletion and setting missing values to the mean, each of which can lead to bias and false identification of significant differences (Croy & Novins, 2005). The MI technique was developed based on the seminal work of Rubin (1987) (for a recent and accessible discussion regarding the use of multiple imputation and other methods for missing variables see work by Croy & Novins, 2005).

MI is performed by creating multiple databases based on observed values. In the study five fully imputed databases were created. Analyses were performed separately in each imputed dataset, and the final point estimates reported in the results are a statistical average of the results of analyses carried out with each of the datasets individually. Standard errors are calculated using an (Analysis of Variance) ANOVA-like formula that accounts for both sampling variation within modelled datasets as well as variability among datasets that reflects the models' uncertainty. The study utilized Royston's (2004) MICE (multiple imputation by chained equations) procedure to impute each of the datasets. This procedure employs switching regression, an iterative multivariable regression technique. UVIS (univariate imputation sampling) is called multiple times by MICE to impute missing values for each specified variable based on a multiple regression model using specified predictors. Micombine commands are then used to produce model estimates incorporating the ANOVA-like procedure to produce reasonable standard errors.

The variables with the most missing data included number of mental health outpatient visits (20.73%), caseworkers' assessment of whether or not the child needed mental health services (8.66%) and the caseworkers' assessment of the level of harm from maltreatment experienced by the child (8.66%). All variables included in the analysis with missing data were imputed.

We used a propensity score matching technique to estimate the effect of outpatient mental health services on internalizing and externalizing problems at 18-month follow-up. Propensity scores are used to produce an estimate of the effect of a treatment by creating a comparison group matched on potentially confounding covariates. These covariates must either be measured before the treatment, or arguably be unaffected by the treatment. In this study, the treatment is the receipt of outpatient mental health services. The first step of analysis included the use of baseline covariates to create balanced groups that are highly similar on all variables except in that the treatment group received outpatient mental health services and the comparison group did not.

Stata's psmatch2 command was used to create the balanced groups. If good balance is achieved on all covariates, then any differences between the two groups can arguably be attributed to the effect of treatment. Balance was first achieved by using the first implicate to construct an optimal model. Multiple propensity score models were tested for balance before the final model, which evidenced the best overall balance, was used to estimate the treatment effect. The final propensity score matching model was applied to each of the implicates and weights were created in each to reflect the number of times each observation was matched in the final model using Stata's micombine command. We addressed further remaining imbalance between matched groups by using additional covariance adjustment to produce the estimated treatment effect in the final model.

The impact of outpatient mental health services for children in foster care

The unweighted sample characteristics of the children included in this study are presented in Table 2.1. Although the mean behavioral problems score on the CBCL falls below the clinical level for this sample, caseworkers indicated that they believed that over half of the children are in need of mental health services. However, only about a quarter of the children received outpatient mental health services over the course of the 18 months of the study.

The balance statistics for the propensity score matching model are presented in Table 2.2. The 'unmatched' means and percentages presented in this table represent the characteristics of the sample when those who have received outpatient mental health services are simply compared to those who have not received outpatient mental health services without matching. For example, before matching, children who received outpatient mental health services had a mean baseline externalizing problems CBCL score of 60.55 and those children who did not receive services had a mean score of 57.26. After matching the groups using the propensity scores the groups are more similar with scores of 60.55 versus 59.37, respectively. In some cases balance was greatly improved for the covariates including caseworker's perception of need, sexual abuse history, and days in current placement. Overall, good balance was achieved in most of the covariates. Only the 'other maltreatment' (i.e. children who suffered maltreatment that could not be classified as physical abuse, sexual abuse, or neglect) covariate

Table 2.1 Unweighted sample characteristics (n = 439)

			n	Percentage of mean	SE or SD
Treatment					
	*Outpatient mental health use		144	.26	.03
Baseline covariates					
	*Externalising CBCL scores baseline			57.40	1.21
	*Internalising CBCL score baseline			54.03	1.37
	*Caseworker perceived need for care		246	.56	.03
Sociodemographic characteristics					
	Child age			7.62	.27
	Child gender (Male=1)		228	.52	.05
	Child race/ethnicity				
		Black	180	.41	.05
		White	154	.35	.05
		Hispanic	75	.17	.03
		Other	31	.07	.05
	*Government support		171	.39	.03
Maltreatment					
	Physical abuse		26	.06	.01
	Sexual abuse		31	.07	.02
	Neglect		250	.57	.04
	Other		132	.30	.03
	Level of harm			3.20	.08
Foster care					
	Kin care		162	.37	.04
	Days in current placement			597.63	48.29
	*Caregiver high school education		373	.85	.03

*For those values with missing data where multiple imputation was employed, the number of children in each category is an estimate derived from the model predicted percentage.

approached a statistically significant difference between the treatment and control group.

Table 2.3 presents the final propensity score model estimate with additional covariance adjustment. Use of outpatient mental health services had no statistically significant impact on either externalizing or internalizing behavior problems. The only covariate that was statistically significant in the model despite the balance between the two groups was the baseline externalizing and internalizing standardized scores for the externalizing and internalizing models, respectively. Each of the baseline scores was significant at the $p < = 0.000$ level in predicting outcomes at 18-month follow-up.

Table 2.2 Propensity score matching balance statistics (n = 120 treatment, n = 92 comparison)

Covariate		Percentage or mean Treated	Percentage or mean Control	Covariate		Percentage or mean Treated	Percentage or mean Control
externalising problems	Unmatched	60.55	57.26	Physical abuse	Unmatched	.13	.14
	Matched	60.55	59.37		Matched	.13	.12
Internalising problems	Unmatched	57.47	54.36	Sexual abuse	Unmatched	.11	.04
	Matched	57.47	55.59		Matched	.11	.12
Caseworker perceived need	Unmatched	.64	.51	Neglect	Unmatched	.46	.55
	Matched	.64	.64		Matched	.46	.56
Age	Unmatched	8.46	7.16	Other maltreatment*	Unmatched	.31	.27
	Matched	8.46	9.16		Matched	.31	.21
Male	Unmatched	.49	.51	Level of harm	Unmatched	3.16	3.24
	Matched	.49	.41		Matched	3.16	3.23
Black	Unmatched	.43	.46	Days in current placement	Unmatched	512.60	540.94
	Matched	.43	.42		Matched	512.60	527.70
Hispanic	Unmatched	.18	.16	Kin caregiver	Unmatched	.33	.33
	Matched	.18	.11		Matched	.33	.29
Other	Unmatched	.43	.46	Caregiver high school education	Unmatched	.85	.86
	Matched	.43	.42		Matched	.85	.85
White	Unmatched	.32	.32	Caregiver income support	Unmatched	.38	.46
	Matched	.32			Matched	.38	.42

*Nearing statistical significance p<=.10.

Table 2.3 Effect of outpatient mental health on behaviour problems at 18-month follow-up propensity score matching model estimate with covariance adjustment (n = 212)

		Externalising		Internalising	
		b	SE	b	SE
Treatment		2.85	2.25	1.87	1.93
	Outpatient mental health use				
Baseline covariates					
	Externalising CBCL scores baseline	.51***	.09	−.05***	.12
	Internalising CBCL score baseline	.00	.09	.52	.11
	Caseworker perceived need for care	.17	1.95	2.79	2.24
	Child black	.15	3.18	1.50	3.20
	Child Hispanic	−1.42	3.48	−1.60	3.83
	Child white	2.18	3.34	3.02	3.65
	Child gender (male=1)	−1.42	1.68	−1.12	.28
	Child age	.24	.22	−.08	2.74
	Government support	.34	2.01	−1.12	2.62
	Caregiver high school education	1.87	2.33	1.63	1.23
	Maltreatment harm	−.60	1.00	−.06	1.84
	Kin care	−2.23	1.71	−2.58	00
	Days in current placement	.00	.00	.00	3.45
	Physical abuse	4.67	2.88	1.49	4.27
	Sexual abuse	−.01	3.69	3.13	2.77
	Neglect	2.44	2.34	2.90	9.05
	Constant	24.40	8.42	21.71	

Child other race/ethnicity and other form of maltreatment are the reference groups.
***p<=.001 level.

Implications for children in foster care who receive outpatient mental health services

The present study findings suggest that outpatient mental health services provided to children who have experienced long-term foster care in the United States do not result in any improvement in children's behavioral health. In reality, little is known about the type and quality of mental health services child welfare involved youth receive nationwide. The few studies that do exist suggest that children are not receiving outpatient mental health services proven to be effective in reducing children's behavior problems (Kolko, 2006; McKay et al., 2004). Instead, youth frequently receive untested treatments with questionable effectiveness. Unfortunately, this issue pervades not only in child welfare and foster care, but across the larger child and adolescent mental health system as well. Despite the increasing availability of a number of evidence-based interventions with demonstrated efficacy in reducing behavioral problems among child welfare populations, many of these interventions have not been widely implemented in practice (Garland, Hawley, Brookman-Frazee, & Hurlburt, 2008; Hurlburt et al., 2007; Kazdin, 2004). Given the tremendous mental health need of foster children and the volume of services purchased by the child welfare agencies, current policy and practice efforts must focus on ensuring that child welfare involved youth have access to effective mental health interventions.

The strengths of this study included the use of a nationally representative sample of children who have experienced long-term foster care. We also made a systematic effort to parse out the effect of receiving outpatient mental health services from key confounding covariates by using propensity score matching. Propensity score matching is a useful method for estimating the impact of services, like outpatient mental health use, which cannot be easily tested through randomized controlled trials. The model is preferable over traditional regression analyses because it provides an opportunity to critically examine and improve the comparability of the treatment and control groups by using diagnostic statistics before estimating the treatment effect.

We also acknowledge the limitations of the study. If the matched treatment and control groups differ from one another on important covariates, then the assumptions that underlie the propensity score matching technique may be compromised. The two groups should be arguably equal with the exception of one factor: whether or not they received the outpatient mental health services. Using the balance statistics as a diagnostic tool, there may have been a balance problem on the type of maltreatment. The difference between the treatment and control groups neared statistical significance on this covariate. The children who received outpatient treatment were more likely to have experienced some form of maltreatment that could not be classified as physical abuse, sexual abuse, or neglect. Some examples of these other forms of maltreatment include emotional maltreatment and exploitation. Despite some imbalance, overall, relatively good balance on key covariates that have consistently been linked to children's use of mental health services and behavioral health outcomes was achieved in this study including baseline behavioral health and placement stability. In addition, the use of additional covariance adjustment further addresses any remaining imbalance between the treatment and control groups.

As with many large-scale datasets, there is often a trade-off between the breadth and the depth of measures that are collected. In this case there are no measures of certain key indicators related to the quality and duration of service use. Some children may access high-quality outpatient services, while others do not. Similarly we cannot pinpoint the exact timing of the outpatient mental health treatment across the 18 months of the study. Some children may have begun service use some time between baseline and follow-up, while others were continuing ongoing service use. Still others may have ended and begun service in the same time frame. However, by defining treatment as having at least three outpatient mental health visits, we have some protection against including children who have only just begun outpatient mental health services, or had only a single visit.

Limitations notwithstanding, the study provided evidence that children in long-term foster care are not receiving adequate mental health prevention and intervention services. As previous studies have demonstrated, children in long-term foster care have greater mental health service needs, and greater mental health service utilization (Burns et al., 2004; Landsverk, Slymen, & Leslie, 2004) than children in the general population. Yet, the quality of these services has been frequently documented as ineffective. This may be due to various mental health service delivery problems ranging from poor client engagement to lax intervention fidelity (Kolko, 2006; McKay, et al., 2004). Future research regarding outpatient mental health service use among children in out-of-home care would be strengthened by the inclusion of more detailed information regarding the timing and nature of service use. In particular, research is needed to guide the implementation and maintenance of high-quality mental health services for children in foster care. As evidence-based interventions increasingly permeate throughout the mental health system, special attention should be paid to the effectiveness of treatments for children in out-of-home care as these children represent one of the largest and most vulnerable populations served by the mental health care system.

Note

1 A version of this chapter was previously published as: Bellamy, J., Traube, D., & Gopalan, G. (2010). A national study of the impact of outpatient mental health services for children in long-term foster care. *Clinical Child Psychology and Psychiatry*, 15(4), 467–480.

References

Aarons, G.A., James, S., Monn, A.R., Raghavan, R., Wells, R., & Leslie, L. (2010). 'Behavior problems and placement change in a national child welfare sample: A prospective study'. *Journal of the American Academy of Child & Adolescent Psychiatry*, 49(1), 70–80.

Achenbach, T.M. (1991). *Integrative Guide for the 1991 CBCL14-18, YSR, and TRF Profiles*. Burlington: University of Vermont, Department of Psychiatry.

Ascher, B.H., Farmer, E.M.Z., Burns, B.J., & Angold, A. (1996). 'The Child and Adolescent Services Assessment (CASA): Description and psychometrics'. *Journal of Emotional and Behavioral Disorders*, 4, 12–20.

Administration for Children & Families [ACF]. (2005). *CPS sample component wave 1 data analysis report*. Administration for Children & Families.

Becker, M., Jordon, N., & Larsen, R. (2006). 'Behavioral health service use and costs among children in foster care'. *Child Welfare*, 85(3), 633–647.

Bickman, L., Smith, C.M., Lambert, E.W., & Andrade, A.R. (2003). 'Evaluation of a congressionally mandated wraparound demonstration'. *Journal of Child and Family Studies*, 12(2), 135–156.

Bradley, B., Westen, D., Mercer, K.B., Binder, E.B., Jovanovic, T., et al. (2011). 'Association between childhood maltreatment and adult emotional dysregulation in a low-income, urban, African American sample: Moderation by oxytocin receptor gene'. *Development and Psychopathology*, 23(2), 439–452.

Buehler, C., Rhodes, K.W., Orme, & Cuddeback, G. (2006). 'The potential for successful family foster care: Conceptualizing competency domains for foster parents'. *Child Welfare*, 85(3), 523–58.

Burns, B.J., Phillips, S.D., Wagner, H.R., Barth, R.P., Kolko, D.J., Campbell, Y., et al. (2004). 'Mental health need and access to mental health services by youths involved with child welfare: A national survey'. *Journal of the American Academy of Child and Adolescent Psychology*, 43, 960–970.

Cicchetti, D. & Toth, S. L. (2004). 'Child maltreatment'. *Annual Review of Clinical Psychology*, 1, 409–438.

Cox, M.E., Orme, J.G., & Rhodes, K.W. (2003). 'Willingness to foster children with emotional or behavioral problems'. *Journal of Social Service Research*, 29(4), 23–51.

Croy, C.D. & Novins, D.K. (2005). 'Methods for addressing missing data in psychiatric and developmental research'. *Journal of the American Academy of Adolescent and Child Psychiatry*, 44(12), 1230–1240.

Cuddeback, G.S. (2004). 'Kinship family foster care: A methodological and substantive synthesis of research'. *Children and Youth Services Review*, 26, 623–639.

Farmer, E.M.Z., Angold A., Burns, B.J., & Costello, E.J. (1994). 'Reliability of self-reported service use: Test-retest consistency of children's responses to the Child and Adolescent Services Assessment (CASA)'. *Journal of Child and Family Studies*, 3, 307–325.

Garland, A.F., Hawley, K.M., Brookman-Frazee, L., & Hurlburt, M.S. (2008). 'Identifying common elements of evidence-based psychosocial treatments for children's disruptive behavior problems'. *Journal of the American Academy of Child & Adolescent Psychiatry*, 47, 505–514.

Geen, R., Sommers, A., & Cohen, M. (2005). *Medicaid spending on foster children*. The Urban Institute Brief No. 2, August 2005. Retrieved on 7/11/12 from http://www.urban.org/UploadedPDF/311221_medicaid_spending.pdf

Hurlburt, M., Barth, R.P., Leslie, L.K., Landsverk, J.A., & McCrae, J.S. (2007). 'Building on strengths: Current status and opportunities for improvement of parent training for families in child welfare services'. In R. Haskins, F.H. Wulczyn, & M.B. Webb (Eds.), *Child protection: Using research to improve policy and practice* (pp. 81–106). Washington, DC: Brookings.

Kaplow, J.B. & Widom, C.S. (2007). 'Age of onset of child maltreatment predicts long-term mental health outcomes'. *Journal of Abnormal Psychology*, 116(1), 176–187.

Kazdin, A. (2004). 'Evidence-based treatments: challenges and priorities for practice and research'. *Child and Adolescent Psychiatric Clinics of North America*, 13, 923–940.

Keller, T.E., Salazar, A.M., & Courtney, M.E. (2010). 'Prevalence and timing of diagnosable mental health, alcohol, and substance use problems among older adolescents in the child welfare system'. *Children and Youth Services Review*, 32(4), 626–634.

Kerker, B.D. & Dore, M.M. (2006). 'Mental health needs and treatment of foster youth: Barriers and opportunities'. *American Journal of Orthopsychiatry*, 76(1), 138–147.

Kolko, D.J. (2006). 'Commentary: Studying usual care in child and adolescent therapy: It's anything but routine'. *Clinical Psychology: Science and Practice*, 13, 47–52.

Lambert, W. & Bickman, L. (2004). 'The "clock-setting" cure: How children's symptoms might improve after ineffective treatment'. *Child and Adolescent Psychiatry*, 55(4), 381–382.

Landsverk, J., Slymen, D.J. & Leslie, L.K. (2004). 'Predictors of outpatient mental health service use: Role of foster care placement change'. *Mental Health Services Research*, 6, 127–141.
Leathers, S.J., Atkins, M.S., Spielfogel, J.E., McMeel, L.S., Wesley, J.M., & Davis, R. (2009). 'Context-specific mental health services for children in foster care'. *Children Youth Services Review*, doi:10.1016/j.childyouth.2009.05.016.
Leslie, L.K., Gordon, J.N., Meneken, L., Premji, K., Michelmore, K.L., & Ganger, W. (2005a). 'The physical, developmental, and mental health needs of young children in child welfare by initial placement type'. *Developmental and Behavioral Pediatrics*, 26(3), 177–185.
Leslie, L.K., Hurlburt, M.S., James, S., Landsverk, J., Slymen, D., & Zhang, J. (2005b). 'Relationship between entry into child welfare and mental health service use'. *Psychiatric Services* 56, 981–987.
Leslie, L.K., Hurlburt, M.S., Landsverk, J., Barth, R.P., & Slymen, D.J. (2004). 'Outpatient mental health services for children in foster care: A national perspective'. *Child Abuse and Neglect*, 28, 697–712.
Manly, J.T., Cicchetti, D., & Barnett, D. (1994). 'The impact of subtype, frequency, chronicity, and severity of child maltreatment on social competence and behaviour problems'. *Development and Psychology*, 6, 121–143.
McKay, M.M., Hibbert, R., Hoagwood, K., Rodriguez, J., Murray, L., & Legerksi, J. (2004). 'Integrating evidence-based engagement interventions into "real world" child mental health settings'. *Brief Treatment and Crisis Intervention*, 4, 177–186.
McMillen, J.C., Zima, B., Scott, L., Ollie, M., Munson, M.R., & Spitznagel, E. (2004). 'The mental health service use of older youth in foster care'. *Psychiatric Services*, 55(7), 811–817.
Oshri, A., Rogosch, F.A., Burnette, M.L., & Cicchetti, D. (2011). 'Developmental pathways to adolescent cannabis abuse and dependence: child maltreatment, emerging personality, and internalizing versus externalizing psychopathology'. *Psychology of Addictive Behaviors*, 25(4), 634–644.
Raghavan, R., Zima, B.T., Andersen, R.M., Leibowitz, A.A., Schuster, M.A., & Landsverk, J. (2005). 'Psychotropic medication use in a national probability sample of children in the child welfare system'. *Journal of Child and Adolescent Psychopharmacology*, 15, 97–106.
Royston, P. (2004). 'Multiple imputation of missing values'. *Stata Journal*, 4, 227–241.
Rubin, D.B. (1987). *Multiple imputation for non-response in surveys*. New York: Wiley.
Springer, K.W., Sheridan, J., Kuo, D., & Carnes, M. (2007). 'Long term physical and mental health consequences of childhood physical abuse: Results from a large population-based sample of men and women'. *Child Abuse & Neglect*, 31(5), 517–530.
StataCorp. 2007. *Stata Statistical Software: Release 10*. College Station, TX: StataCorp LP.
Stahmer, A.C., Leslie, L.K., Hurlburt, M., Barth, R.P., Webb, M.B., & Landsverk, J. (2005). 'Developmental and behavioral needs and service use for young children in child welfare'. *Pediatrics*, 116, 890–900.
Stiffman, A.R., Pescosolido, B., & Cabassa, L.J. (2004). 'Building a model to understand youth service access: The Gateway Provider Model'. *Mental Health Services Research*, 6, 189–198.
Strijker, J., Zandberg, T., & van der Meulen, B.F. (2005). 'Typologies and outcomes for foster children'. *Child & Youth Care Forum*, 34(1), 43–55.

Tarren-Sweeney, M. (2010). 'Concordance of mental health impairment and service utilization among children in care'. *Clinical Child Psychology & Psychiatry*, 15, 481.

Xinsheng, Kaiser, A.P. & Hancock, T.B. (2004). 'Parent and teacher agreement on child behaviour checklist items in a sample of preschoolers from low-income and predominantly African American families'. *Journal of Clinical Child and Adolescent Psychology*, 33(2), 303–312.

3 Our twenty-first century quest

Locating effective mental health interventions for children and young people in care, and those adopted from care

Michael Tarren-Sweeney

The rationale for providing mental health services to children in care, and those subsequently adopted, ultimately depends on the availability of mental health interventions that are meaningfully effective *for them*. Yet, among clinicians who work with these children, there is reasonable consensus that standard psychological and pharmacological interventions appear less effective for them. Empirical support for this observation is reported in Chapter 2 by Jennifer Bellamy and her colleagues. They carried out an analysis of the effects of standard out-patient mental health treatment for a representative population sample of clinic-referred children in long-term foster care, drawn from the US National Survey of Child and Adolescent Well-being (NSCAW). They found that outpatient treatment had no independent effect on 18-month changes to caregiver-reported CBCL scores, suggesting that collectively at least, interventions that constitute standard outpatient treatment in the US may not be effective over this timeframe.

Yet, there is an increasing expectation that clinicians and mental health services working with children in care and adopted children should employ *evidence-based interventions* for treatment of disorders commonly diagnosed among these groups of children (Barth, Crea, John, Thoburn, & Quinton, 2005). With this in mind, the present chapter considers the availability, relevance and strength of evidence about the effectiveness of mental health interventions offered to this book's target populations – and proposes a way forward for future effectiveness research. Throughout the chapter, the term 'mental health interventions' refers to those that directly involve children and young people, as well as those that seek to indirectly effect therapeutic change through caregiver training, counselling and support.

The current status of mental health interventions for children in care and those adopted from care

When considering the effectiveness of mental health interventions for referred children in care and adopted children, it is important to keep in mind that they are not a clinically homogenous group. At the very least, we need to separately consider treatment effectiveness for two broad clinical sub-populations (see Chapter 1 for more detail), namely:

- Those children who have relatively non-complex psychopathology that can be reasonably formulated as discrete mental disorders or co-morbidity using standard diagnostic classification (around 35% of the CICS cohort); and
- Those children who present with complex attachment- and trauma-related psychopathology that is not adequately conceptualised within standard classification (around 20% of the CICS cohort) (Tarren-Sweeney, In Press).

Whereas evidence gathered on the effectiveness of diagnosis-specific interventions from clinical trials with children at large have some relevance for the first group listed above, it is unreasonable to infer that such evidence can be generalised to the second group.

Types of mental health interventions

Mental health interventions are usually grouped according to the theoretical frameworks that guided their development, such as *behavioural, cognitive behavioural, psychodynamic*, and *systemic* psychotherapies. This approach is not particularly useful for the present purpose, for two reasons. Firstly, for this population we need to increasingly focus on multi-systemic interventions that necessarily involve therapeutic mechanisms explained by multiple developmental theories, particularly social learning, attachment, and systems theories. Secondly, many of the interventions that are proposed to involve a specific theorised mechanism are more likely to stimulate additional (even unintended) therapeutic mechanisms when they are employed in foster and adoptive families. Instead, I think it is more useful to group mental health interventions employed in the care and adoption fields into the following categories:

1. Primary prevention interventions provided to children and young people exposed to specific adverse events or circumstances, which are designed to 'inoculate' against the emergence of mental health symptoms, felt insecurity or other adverse developmental outcomes. Two examples of this are sexual abuse counselling provided to children following disclosure of sexual abuse, and life story work carried out with children who have complex care histories and/or disrupted attachments. In some instances these same interventions are prescribed to children after problems begin to emerge.
2. Individual or group psychotherapy targeting specific symptoms, disorders or functioning. These are more commonly employed with older children and young people. Some examples include social skills training, trauma-focused CBT, dialectical behaviour therapy and play therapy. In some

cases individual psychotherapies are adapted to involve carers, without necessarily employing a systemic focus.
3 Systemic family/dyadic psychotherapies that involve two or more individuals from a family or alternate family group. Some examples are family therapy, parent–child psychotherapy, attachment narrative therapy (ANT, described in Chapter 7) (Dallos & Dallos, 2013) and dyadic developmental psychotherapy (Hughes, 2004).
4 Interventions primarily directed towards caregivers, which aim to maximise caregiving as a primary therapeutic mechanism and/or sustain children's placements. Examples include attachment and biobehavioural catchup (Dozier, Bick, & Bernard, 2011), parent–child interaction therapy (Timmer, Urquiza, & Zebell, 2006), enhanced adoptive parenting (EAP, see Chapter 4) (Rushton & Monck, 2009) and generic family behavioural interventions (such as Triple P, and Incredible Years).
5 Multi-systemic/wraparound interventions that target multiple components of a child's developmental ecology. These interventions simultaneously focus on reducing mental health symptoms (especially behavioural difficulties), strengthening close relationships, improving other functional outcomes (e.g. focusing on school education and peer socialisation) and altering children's developmental pathways. The best-known example is multidimensional treatment foster care.

The specificity of interventions for children in care and adopted children

Some interventions are designed specifically for children in care and/or those adopted from care, such as multidimensional treatment foster care for preschoolers (MTFC-P) (Fisher, Burraston, & Pears, 2005), attachment and biobehavioural catchup, and enhanced adoptive parenting. There are also some interventions that have been especially modified or adapted for use with these populations or their caregivers, such as attachment narrative therapy. However, most mental health interventions offered for these children and their carers are neither specifically designed, nor modified for use with them. Sometimes these interventions are matched to children's symptoms or diagnoses, following guidance on evidence-based practice for children at large, without reference to symptom complexity or developmental context. There are few interventions that have been designed or modified to treat complex symptomatology, regardless of children's care status. However, efforts to modify dialectical behaviour therapy and mentalisation-based treatment for use with children and adolescents opens possibilities for more appropriate individual psychotherapies for children who have complex, trait-like symptomatology. Finally, some 'therapeutic' interventions and counselling are provided to children in care and adopted children without reference to a clinical formulation, and without sufficient assessment data. Often this occurs when a therapist is trained in a single method, which they assume

40 *Michael Tarren-Sweeney*

provides therapeutic benefits regardless of the type of difficulties a child presents with, or their developmental context.

Guidance from published reviews

There have been four general reviews of mental health interventions for children and young people in care in recent years (Craven & Lee, 2006; Landsverk, Burns, Stambaugh, & Reutz, 2006, 2009; Leve, et al., 2012; Racusin, Maerlender, Sengupta, Isquith, & Straus, 2005), as well as one relevant commentary (Barth, et al., 2005), but no equivalent reviews for children adopted from care (although Alan Rushton describes several interventions for adoptive families in Chapter 4). These reviews vary somewhat in their methodology, extent of systematic appraisal, how they rate treatment effectiveness, and conclusions.

Aside from published case reports, each of these reviews identified very few treatment studies carried out with children in care. It is notable that a small number of randomised controlled trials (RCTs) have been published more recently, which I describe later in this chapter. In lieu of effectiveness data that are specific to children in care, these reviews largely focus on the evidence base for treatments of 'the most prevalent mental conditions found among children in foster care' (Landsverk, et al., 2009), gathered from RCTs carried out with children at large. Interestingly, these reviews do not question the extent to which such data can be generalised to children in care, and adopted children. Some of the reviews do, however, refer to effectiveness data obtained for maltreated children, which holds greater validity for 'in care' and adopted children. Additionally, there have been several reviews on the effectiveness of specific types or classes of interventions, namely:

- Interventions for foster parents (Dozier, Albus, Fisher, & Sepulveda, 2002; Turner, MacDonald, & Dennis, 2009)
- Attachment-based support services and psychotherapies (Howe, 2006)
- Treatment models for group and residential care (James, 2011)

Guidance from organisations that promote evidence-based practice

Aside from published clinical reviews, clinicians and mental health services obtain guidance from various organisations and services that evaluate or translate the effectiveness of mental health interventions, including professional associations, research clearing houses and organisations whose purpose is to identify and disseminate evidence-based practice – such as the UK's National Institute for Health and Clinical Excellence (NICE). In recent years, a few such organisations have written about the particular mental health needs of children and young people in care (but not children adopted from care) – alluding mainly to the absence of an adequate evidence base, and the need for further clinical effectiveness studies. A recent Faculty of

Child and Adolescent Psychiatry, Royal Australian and New Zealand College of Psychiatrists (RANZCP) report on the mental health needs of children and young people in care, did not examine the effectiveness literature, but instead identified a critical shortfall in 'clinical research into psychological and pharmacological treatment of the complex psychopathology of children in out-of-home care' (Royal Australian & New Zealand College of Psychiatrists, 2008). NICE and the Social Care Institute for Excellence (SCIE) recently published a public health guideline for working with children and young people in care in the UK (NICE & SCIE, 2010). While the guideline neither reviews, nor comments on treatment effectiveness, it recommended that governments should fund and facilitate treatment effectiveness research for this population. Surprisingly, a set of research questions proposed in the guideline exclude any reference to identifying effective mental health interventions for this population – focusing instead on such things as social care models and access to mental health services. NICE has also published a number of clinical guidelines for treatment of child mental health difficulties, some of which are particularly pertinent to 'in care' and adopted children (notably ADHD, PTSD, conduct disorder and depression). However, these guidelines do not examine differential treatment effectiveness for care populations or other vulnerable groups. In general, however, most clinical practice guidelines and treatment reviews published by professional associations to date, have not referred to treatment effectiveness for 'in care' or adopted children – or considered the extent to which efficacy findings generalise to special populations, or to children with complex difficulties, for example, the Australian Psychological Society's review of evidence-based psychological interventions (Australian Psychological Society, 2010).

Presently, the most authoritative guidance on mental health interventions for child welfare clients (including those residing in care and those adopted from care) is provided by the California Evidence-based Clearinghouse for Child Welfare (funded by the state child welfare department). The clearinghouse reviews the effectiveness of mental health interventions in terms of:

- *Scientific rating*: based on classical efficacy/effectiveness data from clinical trials. The scientific rating has a five-point scale, ranging from 'I. well-supported by research evidence', to 'V. concerning practice'; and
- *Child welfare system relevance level*: the extent to which the intervention is either purposely designed for child welfare clients, and/or has been trialled with child welfare samples. Child welfare system relevance levels are *high*, *medium* or *low*.

Findings from clinical treatment trials

As mentioned previously in this chapter, there has been little substantive research into the effectiveness and appropriateness of mental health interventions for children in care and adopted children, either through examining therapy process or therapeutic outcomes. This is not to say that interventions for these populations have not been developed, or that they are ineffective. Rather, most promising interventions have yet to be adequately evaluated. In this section, research findings from five interventions that have been evaluated in clinical trials are summarised and discussed.

Multidimensional treatment foster care

Multidimensional treatment foster care (MTFC) is an intensive, wraparound, multi-component intervention in which children and young people reside for a limited time period with a *treatment* foster family (Chamberlain, 2003). It was initially developed as an alternative to residential and group care for adolescent young offenders and those with severe behavioural and emotional problems, and to date has largely been studied with participants who otherwise would be placed in residential treatment (MacDonald & Turner, 2008). As such, it presents as a particularly promising intervention for young people in the care system whose disruptiveness generates placement instability, who have complex mental health difficulties, and who otherwise are more likely to be placed in residential care. The first research trial of MTFC with older children and young people in care was recently carried out in the UK, involving parallel RCT and observational studies, with most participants being enrolled in the latter study (aged 11–16, N = 219) (Biehal, et al., 2012). Propensity score matching was employed to adjust for differences between the quasi-experimental and control (usual foster care) samples. Importantly, the treatment and control samples were young people who had unstable placement histories, and who had either been in residential care or were on a pathway to residential care. Following propensity score matching, participants who received MTFC did not significantly differ from the control group on a range of outcomes, including subsequent placement stability, participation in education, or recorded offending, and pre-post changes in global functioning (CGAS) and mental health (CBCL, SDQ, HoNOSCA, DAWBA-AD) (Biehal, et al., 2012). Young people who had serious antisocial behaviour problems did better if they resided in MTFC, while those who were not seriously antisocial did better in regular care. It was notable that many of the latter group had mental health difficulties other than antisocial behaviour. These findings suggest that MTFC may be effective for older children and young people in the care system who are seriously antisocial, and who do not have complex mental health difficulties.

Multidimensional treatment foster care for pre-schoolers

Multidimensional treatment foster care for preschoolers (MTFC-P) and early intervention foster care (EIFC) are variations of MTFC adapted for children in care aged 3–6 years, who have yet to obtain permanent placements (Fisher, Gunnar, Chamberlain, & Reid, 2000). It is unclear whether EIFC and MTFC-P differ in any substantial way, or if the intervention that was previously called EIFC was later renamed MTFC-P. Whereas MTFC is designed for children with existing mental health difficulties, MTFC-P is a preventative, population-based intervention for pre-school-aged children in care. The MTFC-P contains a number of developmentally informed variations from MTFC that make it more appropriate for preschool-aged children. The 'intervention is delivered via a team approach to the child, foster care provider, and permanent placement resource (birth parents and adoptive relatives or non-relatives)' (Fisher, et al., 2005). A goal of the intervention is to transition children to a permanent placement, typically involving 6 to 9 months (Fisher, et al., 2005).

An RCT carried out by the intervention developers[1] demonstrated several important findings that suggest MTFC-P is an efficacious intervention for such children. Compared with pre-schoolers residing in regular temporary foster care (the control intervention), children placed with MTFC-P caregivers showed significant increases in secure attachment behaviour and reductions in insecure avoidant attachment behaviour over the study period (Fisher & Kim, 2007). By the end of the treatment period, they also manifested stress hormone activity patterns resembling that of non-maltreated children at large, whereas the control sample continued to show abnormal stress hormone activity consistent with their early history of maltreatment (Fisher, et al., 2000). Among a sub-sample of children who entered the study with unstable placement histories (N = 52), children in a MTFC-P placement had double the rate of retention within their subsequent permanent placements two years post-study, than control children (Fisher, Kim, & Pears, 2009). Except for the stability of subsequent permanent placements, these effects were measured whilst the participants were in the care of their treatment and regular foster parents. Otherwise, the effects of children being moved to a subsequent placement, including any effects of loss of attachment figures, could not be measured using this particular study design, as both the treatment and control samples experienced a subsequent change of placement.

MTFC-P is a particularly promising intervention for young children with mental health difficulties and prior placement instability, who would otherwise have required a further temporary placement prior to obtaining permanency. It perhaps has the potential to stabilise children in such circumstances, and to increase their chances of attaining non-disrupted permanent care. Given such demonstrated benefits, I think it is important to guard against seeing MTFC-P as necessary preparation for permanency for young children in care who have serious behaviour problems, if the implication is that their time in temporary foster care is extended (see discussion about the developmental appropriateness of extended temporary care at the end of this chapter).

44   Michael Tarren-Sweeney

Keep

Whereas MTFC and MTFC-P involve active placement of a single child or young person with specially trained treatment foster parents (with no other child residing in the home), elements of MTFC have also been modified and applied as a more naturalistic intervention designed to support existing foster and kinship placements, called KEEP (keeping foster and kinship parents trained and supported) (Price, Chamberlain, Landsverk, & Reid, 2009). KEEP is a less radical intervention than MTFC for many children already residing in care because it does not require a change of placement when treatment is completed, and it is also designed to support placements that have more than one child. Therefore, KEEP can be offered without disrupting existing relationships with long-term or permanent caregivers and co-placed siblings.

The effectiveness of the KEEP intervention has been evaluated in a large RCT that compared outcomes for children in foster and kinship care (aged 5–12 years, N = 700) randomly allocated to either the KEEP programme or to continue receiving standard casework services (that included some training for carers) (Price, et al., 2009). It is unclear whether this study measured access to other mental health services or interventions by control children during the study period. Children whose caregivers received the KEEP intervention showed a modest, though meaningful pre-post intervention reduction in their mean number of behaviour problems per day (reduced from 5.9 to 4.4), whereas the group who received usual care showed less meaningful reduction (5.8 to 5.4) (Chamberlain, et al., 2008). Furthermore, the biggest reductions in behaviour problems were observed among those children who had higher levels of initial problems. The other critical finding was that children in the KEEP supported placements were more likely to obtain a planned move to a permanent placement (i.e. restoration, permanent kinship placement or adoption) than control children (Price, et al., 2008). However, there was no difference between the groups in the rate of unplanned placement breakdowns and other negative exits from children's current placements.

Attachment and biobehavioural catchup (ABC)

The ABC intervention was developed by Mary Dozier and her colleagues to facilitate relationship formation and associated biobehavioural developmental for maltreated infants and toddlers, and for those who have experienced disrupted attachments. The intervention was evaluated in an RCT with a sample of infants and toddlers in foster care, where the control intervention was provision of developmental education. Published findings were derived from a number of different analyses carried out at different stages of participant recruitment, with the number of study participants ranging from 46 to 93, with half of those numbers being randomly allocated to each of the ABC and control interventions. In the first analysis, treatment infants (N = 23) showed significantly less avoidant attachment behaviour than control infants following distress-eliciting incidents reported over a three-day period (Dozier, et al., 2009). However, this analysis does not appear to take into account infants' pre-treatment attachment security. In the second set of analyses, the distribution of post-intervention morning and afternoon cortisol production by treatment infants (N = 30) closely paralleled that of a comparison sample of infants at large who were not in foster care (N = 104), and was significantly lower than that produced by control infants (Dozier, et al., 2006). Moreover, the difference in mean cortisol production between treatment and control infants was developmentally significant. While treatment and control infants manifested a similar scale of post-intervention behaviour problems, an age effect was found among the treatment sample – with treated toddlers (18–36 months) having fewer behaviour problems than treated infants. In the third set of analyses, treatment infants (N = 46) showed considerably lower stress reactions than control infants during a strange situation procedure, as measured by cortisol production (measured before, and then 15 and 30 minutes after the procedure) (Dozier, Peloso, Lewis, Laurenceau, & Levine, 2008). An important additional finding was that infants receiving the ABC intervention had very similar cortisol levels at each point of measurement to an additional comparison sample (N = 48) of infants at large who were not in foster care, suggesting their stress regulation is normatively distributed.

In summary, there is good evidence that the ABC intervention has a therapeutic effect on the stress regulation and attachment security of infants and toddlers in care, but inconclusive evidence that this translates into reduced behaviour problems shortly after treatment. It is important to note that achieving normalisation of infant stress regulation and increased attachment security has far greater developmental significance for subsequent mental health, than reducing their frequency of behaviour problems.

Comparison of three trauma symptom interventions

The effectiveness of three age-bounded interventions designed to treat traumatic stress symptoms was evaluated in a clinical trial with 133 children and young people (aged 3–18) enrolled in a wraparound foster care programme in the United States, who had previously experienced a moderate or severely traumatic incident (Weiner, Schneider, & Lyons, 2009). The interventions were child–parent psychotherapy (CPP, N = 65, aged 3–6), trauma-focused cognitive behavioural therapy (TF-CBT, N = 35, aged 3–16) and structured psychotherapy for adolescents responding to chronic stress (SPARCS, N = 33, aged 13–18). The goal of CPP is to facilitate young (aged 0–5) children's recovery from traumatic stress by increasing parental sensitivity, strengthening parent–child attachments and boosting children's felt security, using a dyadic psychotherapy format. The extent of children's direct engagement in

CPP varies according to their age. TF-CBT attempts to reduce children's unpleasant physiological trauma symptoms using a range of cognitive, behavioural and psycho-education techniques. While the child is the primary participant in TF-CBT, the intervention includes education for parents that seeks to normalise their child's experiences, moderate unhelpful parental reactions to their child's distress and to provide emotional support for their child. SPARCS is a group intervention for adolescents who have been exposed to traumatic stressors. It employs various components of dialectical behaviour therapy, with strong focus on acquiring improved mindfulness, interpersonal skills and coping abilities. Each of these interventions had previously been evaluated with traumatised children at large.

The study design did not include a control intervention, although inclusion of three study interventions provided opportunity to compare their relative effectiveness. The study's primary goal was to identify the relative effectiveness of these interventions with different racial groups. Treatment effect sizes were not reported for the aggregate samples, and some of the ethnicity-treatment groups had too few participants to estimate treatment effectiveness. Clinically meaningful pre-post reductions in trauma symptoms were measured for young African-American, Biracial and Hispanic (but not White) children who received CPP. Clinically meaningful reductions were measured for African-American and White children who received TF-CBT (no other ethnicity group had sufficient sample size). African-American youth who participated in the SPARCS intervention showed a statistically significant, though less clinically meaningful reduction in trauma symptoms (other ethnic groups had insufficient sample size). These results were achieved in a real-world setting, and thus can be considered to be measures of effectiveness. The study findings suggest that CPP and TF-CBT are possibly effective interventions for treatment of trauma symptoms experienced by children in care, while SPARCS is a less promising intervention for young people in care.

Setting the bar higher – what information do we need to establish the effectiveness of mental health interventions for children with complex attachment- and trauma-related difficulties?

Most readers will know that a culture and ideas battle is underway within our clinical professions and workplaces, around what kinds of knowledge we should use to guide our practice; how much weight we place on research findings about the effectiveness of psychological interventions; what parameters should define effectiveness and how they should be measured; and most contentious of all – what constitutes an evidence-based intervention. Many of us have signed up to the underlying principle of evidence-based practice (EBP) – that our clinical work should be guided by the best available evidence. Where we mostly disagree, is on what constitutes 'best available evidence'. The conventional view is that this battle of ideas is driven by opposing epistemological positions – *positivist, empirical science* versus the belief that effective psychotherapy requires *clinical experience and knowledge* that eludes quantification, measurement and 'manualisation'. It is also rooted in a division between the research laboratory and the clinic, as well as a much earlier battle of ideas between behaviourism and psychoanalysis. One's leaning towards these opposing positions is partly a consequence of being socialised within different professional traditions, and for some, in which university programme you were trained. It doesn't help that the principles of EBP are sometimes fervently (mindlessly?) enforced on CAMHS and other clinical services as a form of intellectual hegemony.

Most of us, however, can learn to lean another way if we are presented with compelling, contrary evidence. Many clinicians are struggling to reconcile these opposing views within their own work, rather than holding an unwavering ideological position – clinicians who Nick Midgley describes as *adapters* (Midgley, 2009). Driving this is a disconnect between the principles of working from an empirical evidence base, and the enormous complexity of human psychological development and morbidity – much of which is not yet adequately measured or conceptualised. What continues to fuel this ideas war is that both viewpoints are partially correct – and both are partially blinkered. Importantly, these differences can, and should be reconciled, at least to a point where most of us can come to some agreement.

Most evidence ratings, for example those published in NICE clinical guidelines and in Cochrane systematic reviews, are based on a *hierarchy* of evidence. Within such hierarchies, published case reports are deemed to represent very low evidence (or are not considered to represent evidence at all), while the highest evidence rating is given to interventions that show reasonable treatment effect across several well-designed RCTs, preferably in real-world clinical settings. Those interventions that have only been shown to demonstrate a treatment effect under optimal research conditions (often with carefully selected participants who have very discrete symptomatology) are deemed to be *efficacious*, rather than effective. Clinical trials without an adequate control group, RCTs with small sample size or other methodological weaknesses, comparative effectiveness research (pragmatic trials), and multiple baseline single case designs lie between these two extremes on an evidence hierarchy.

Evidence is also largely rated on the extent and persistence of changes in symptom prevalence and severity, and other relevant outcomes such as social and educational functioning and parental burden of care. Importantly, in terms of how interventions are rated, little weight has been given to research on: therapy process (e.g. what are the therapeutic mechanisms); investigating the contextual factors that optimise or hinder effectiveness; investigation of possible harmful effects (e.g. carrying out post-trial research with those children who show pre-post deterioration, and with early drop-outs); accounting for children's or parents' experience of therapy; long-term alteration to children's developmental pathways; or evidence of neuro-developmental change.

To date, there is remarkably little evidence that existing mental health interventions are effective for children with complex attachment- and trauma-related difficulties. This is not to say that there are no effective interventions. Rather, the present standards with which we rate psychotherapy are disconnected from the reality of assisting children with complex difficulties in real-world clinical settings. Not enough relevant or well-designed research is being carried out, partly I suspect because psychotherapies are too often afforded evidence-based status prematurely (i.e. researchers and funding bodies are not incentivised to work beyond the present evidence standards), and partly because psychotherapy researchers have not understood the importance of measuring and understanding the developmental and psychosocial mechanisms that underlie both children's psychopathology and therapeutic recovery.

In light of this I propose three broad remedies for future development of mental health interventions for children and young people in care, and those adopted from care:

1. Replace existing *evidence hierarchies* with multiple evidence requirements;
2. *Increase the robustness* of psychotherapy randomised controlled trials; and
3. Psychotherapy development and evaluation need to be informed by *adequate conceptualisation and measurement of complex attachment- and trauma-related difficulties*, their *developmental underpinnings*, and the *context of social care systems*

The remainder of this chapter sets out a rationale and framework for each of these broad remedies.

First remedy – replace existing evidence hierarchies with multiple evidence requirements

I believe that mental health intervention evidence ratings should be based on multiple evidence requirements, rather than evidence hierarchies, particularly when evaluating interventions for complex symptomatology. It is useful to compare the standard for rating the effectiveness of psychological treatments with the standard for establishing causality in clinical medicine and public health. Causality is not established from a single *gold standard* form of evidence, but instead, by accumulating *nine* required forms of evidence (strength of association; consistency; specificity; temporal relationship; biological gradient (dose–response relationship); biological plausibility; coherence; experimental evidence; and reasoning by analogy). Thus, a higher standard of evidence is required to establish causality than either treatment efficacy or effectiveness. Interestingly, some of these criteria also seem relevant to establishing the effectiveness of psychological treatments. For example, the specificity criterion refers to isolating causal effects from other influences that may account for a statistical association (i.e. confounding). With interventions, we are similarly interested in measuring the differential effectiveness of clinicians as 'therapists' per se, versus effectiveness that is directly attributable to therapy procedures – as well as interaction effects.

Second remedy – increase the robustness of psychotherapy randomised controlled trials

Well-designed RCTs have exceptional methodological rigour and internal validity. No other research design adequately isolates treatment effects from a myriad of potential biases that create an illusion of effectiveness (Fonagy, Target, Cottrell, Phillips, & Kurtz, 2005). In practice, however, the external validity of psychotherapy RCTs depends on such things as: the conceptual validity of the psychological construct(s) that are the focus of therapy (e.g. is ADHD a valid unitary construct?); the extent to which such construct(s) can be accurately measured or estimated; definitions of meaningful change; the timeframes over which meaningful change should be measured; and the clinical representativeness of psychotherapy and control group participants. A particular challenge for carrying out psychotherapy RCTs (as compared with clinical drug trials for physical morbidity) is accounting for the 'effectiveness' of individual therapists, as distinct from the therapy procedure, especially for those interventions that require a very high level of therapist skill and training. It is extremely difficult to provide adequate control for therapist effectiveness if the control intervention is *treatment as usual*, even in real-world effectiveness trials. Thus, while RCTs employed in psychotherapy research are rigorous, they are presently not sufficiently robust for their findings to translate well to real-world clinical settings. This is especially so for treatment of complex attachment- and trauma-related difficulties.

Listed below, are some suggestions for increasing the robustness of RCTs of mental health interventions for children and young people with complex attachment- and trauma-related difficulties, as well as their families:

Publishing treatment effectiveness metrics that have greater clinical meaning

RCTs typically compare the distributions of pre-post change for the treatment and control groups in quite simple terms, namely effect sizes expressed as standardised group mean score differences (Cohen's *d*) and the statistical significance of the effect size. These data can be compared directly from one RCT to the next, and pooled effect sizes can be calculated from successive

RCTs in a meta-analysis. However, these data are often not clinically meaningful. From a clinical perspective, it is more useful to report the proportions of children in both the treatment and control groups who, during an evaluation timeframe are estimated to show: 1. *clinically meaningful improvement*; 2. *no clinically meaningful change*; and 3. *clinically meaningful deterioration*. This provides a more useful starting point for investigating variables that predict treatment response, as well as variations in response to treatment by clinical and developmental sub-populations (e.g. children who have experienced profound social adversity, children with complex symptomatology).

Employing realistic developmental timeframes for pre-post evaluation

Complex attachment- and trauma-related difficulties (especially those manifested by children exposed to chronic social adversity from an early age) typically follow a long-term developmental course and have trait-like durability. Readers who work with such children will know that their recovery from these difficulties also tends to occur over much longer time periods than does recovery from more discrete, state-like disorders. Among older children who enter care or are adopted with complex difficulties, meaningful therapeutic change is unlikely to be revealed until the child has experienced several years of consistent, structured and sensitive caregiving without a change in caregivers. The implication then is that RCTs with this population need to be set up as long-term studies, providing at least several years of post-treatment assessment. This introduces additional costs and methodological challenges, especially in terms of sample attrition and taking account of other developmental influences on children's mental health and well-being.

Integrating RCTs within larger effectiveness studies

There are methodological and cost advantages in combining various types of effectiveness research within larger studies. An important focus of enquiry is identifying why a treatment is effective for some children, why it is not effective for others, and why it may be harmful for yet others – using a combination of qualitative, epidemiological, neurobiological and clinical research methods. This research potentially yields improvements in psychotherapy procedure, modifications for specific sub-groups, and identifies children and families who are less likely to benefit from an intervention or for whom it may be harmful. A well-designed RCT provides a methodologically superior starting point for carrying out such research. Similarly, integrating RCTs within larger effectiveness studies should provide greater scope for identifying therapeutic mechanisms of change (Kazdin, 2007).

Third remedy – psychotherapy development and evaluation need to be informed by adequate conceptualisation and measurement of complex attachment- and trauma-related difficulties, their developmental underpinnings, and the context of social care systems

Identifying valid constructs and measures

Presently, complex attachment- and trauma-related difficulties are both inadequately conceptualised and poorly measured (DeJong, 2010) (see also Chapter 1). These gaps in our knowledge necessarily compromise research about their treatment. The design and evaluation of mental health interventions with this clinical population will need to employ more sophisticated definitions and measurement of complex difficulties targeted for treatment, than has been the case thus far.

Earlier and more precise indication of developmental recovery

If treatment effectiveness is ultimately measured in terms of meaningful reductions in symptom frequency and severity, but (as explained previously in this chapter) if reductions in complex symptomatology is realistically only attained over relatively long timeframes – then relevant effectiveness research should aim to include fine-grained measures of children's developmental pathways that can identify incremental change, and especially early signs of recovery. Measures of children's stress hormone production have been shown to be more sensitive to therapeutic change over short- to medium-term periods than problem behaviour measures (Dozier, et al., 2008). Further technological advances in the measurement of neurobiological functioning, development of pro-social behaviour measures that are theoretically indicative of early signs of recovery ('green shoots' measures), and the development of qualitative monitoring tools, are needed to adequately evaluate future long-term effectiveness studies of treatments for children in care and adopted children. Small changes can turn out to be pivotal points in the development of a caregiver–child relationship.

The need to design interventions that manipulate complex developmental mechanisms

Complex symptomatology and complex developmental impairment suggests there are multiple mechanisms at work, with likely interaction effects. Understanding the nature and developmental underpinnings of complex symptomatology is made more difficult because we do not yet have a unifying theory of child development. Researchers and clinicians are mostly trained and socialised to make sense of the complexity of human development using relatively simple theoretical frameworks. For example, parenting interventions that are based on principles of social learning theory nonetheless alter qualities of caregiving and caregiver–child relationships that are presently explained by attachment theory. However, neuro-developmental, epidemiological, clinical and behavioural genetics research indicates that the mechanisms and developmental pathways which account for mental ill-health are vastly more complex than what can be explained by present child developmental theory. Yet, most child clinical interventions continue to be primarily guided by relatively simple theoretical frameworks. This needs to change! O'Connor et al. (In Press) recently reported that '*we have found that the parallel paths pursued by social learning theory and attachment theory may be somewhat artificial. There are generalizable effects from treatment, even if there is evidence of distinctiveness from the meditational analyses. Clinical and theoretical progress is most likely where there are further efforts to identify areas of overlap and distinction between these competing models.*' Designing effective interventions for attachment- and trauma-related difficulties will also require an understanding of their proximal causal mechanisms, which are undoubtedly complex (Fonagy & Bateman, 2006; Kazdin, 2007).

Demonstrating the relative cost-effectiveness of long-term multi-faceted interventions

With this in mind, no single 'psychotherapy' is likely to be as effective as employing multiple interventions that operate together on different components of a child's developmental ecology. This reasoning underlies existing multi-component approaches (such as 'wraparound', multi-systemic therapy, and MTFC) that are designed to simultaneously address children's behaviour difficulties, emotional well-being, family relationships, education, self-esteem, etc. I expect that future development of mental health interventions for complex difficulties will necessarily incorporate multiple treatment components. The costs for providing intensive, multifaceted interventions over long timeframes are considerably higher than the costs for providing standard, short-term mental health interventions. Yet the potential economic and social benefits are also considerable. Governments are only likely to support and fund more expensive mental health interventions if there is compelling evidence for their relative cost-effectiveness over standard treatments. Importantly, the economic and social costs of not effecting therapeutic recovery with these populations are considerably higher than those incurred among children in the general population. Along with the need for further clinical treatment research with these populations, there is urgent need for related health economics and health social science research.

Closer monitoring for harmful effects

In contrast to clinical trials of pharmacological mental health treatments, psychotherapy research has largely ignored or side-stepped the question of whether people can be harmed by psychological treatments. By not actively investigating possible indicators of harm (e.g. assessing 'drop out' participants and those whose outcome measures suggest meaningful deterioration), researchers implicitly suggest that the worst psychotherapy outcome is 'no improvement'. Fonagy and Bateman (2006) have speculated that traditional psychotherapies are harmful for some adults with borderline personality disorder (BPD), due to iatrogenic mechanisms involving impaired mentalisation capacity, and the activation of their attachment systems within a therapeutic alliance. Many of the complex attachment- and trauma-related difficulties manifested by young people in care resemble core features of BPD (Tarren-Sweeney, 2013, In Press), suggesting we should be similarly concerned about the potential for psychotherapies to cause them harm. I would argue that ethical research on mental health interventions with these vulnerable populations should necessarily include procedures for monitoring harmful effects.

Cultural enhancement/modification for indigenous and ethnic minority children and families

The most important finding generated from the aforementioned clinical trial of three trauma symptom interventions (Weiner, et al., 2009), was evidence of differential effectiveness of those treatments across different racial groups of children and young people in foster care in the United States. Given that in the western world, indigenous children and children from disadvantaged minority ethnic backgrounds are over-represented within care populations, these findings prompt the need for further research into cultural enhancement/modification of mental health interventions.

The centrality of enduring, loving relationships to mental health recovery and well-being

Multidimensional treatment foster care for preschoolers (MTFC-P) and attachment and biobehavioural catchup (ABC) are designed to counter the developmental effects of pre-care adversity and maltreatment – *as well as* some of the developmental consequences of a flawed model of social care (that creates poor conditions for developing secure attachments, and which delays young children's access to permanent, loving care). MTFC-P is presently applied using a model where young children do not remain with their treatment foster carers (even if they have become attached to them). While some readers will see this as unusual, it should be remembered that MTFC-P is provided within conventional social care systems that pay insufficient regard to the psychosocial effects of impermanent care of infants and young children; and that there is good evidence that MTFC-P is demonstrably preferable to regular temporary foster care.

Ultimately, I believe the therapeutic potential of MTFC-P and ABC would be extended if child welfare jurisdictions were to apply them within a reformed social care system – one that does away with extended periods of non-permanent care for infants and young children. There is no fundamental reason why children's agencies could not implement (or modify) the MTFC-P and ABC interventions within a concurrent planning social care model – reducing the likelihood of children having a planned move to further caregivers after treatment is completed. With concurrent planning, the infant or young child who is in need of care is placed with caregivers who are simultaneously temporary foster parents and prospective adoptive parents, while court assessments, birth parental interventions and final care proceedings are carried out (Monck, Reynolds, & Wigfall, 2004). This model of care is designed to reduce placement changes for young children who are not restored to their parents' care, and offers greater potential for committed, sensitive temporary caregiving for those young children who are restored.

In recent years, some scholars have claimed that the social care field has focused too greatly on attachment theory as a vehicle for therapeutic recovery of children in care, and that this has blinded us to recognising other psychotherapeutic opportunities (Barth, et al., 2005). This has partly come as a response to controversy about both the effectiveness and humaneness of so-called 'attachment therapies' (Chaffin, et al., 2006; Dozier, 2003). In my view, this debate has been overshadowed by the misappropriation of the word 'attachment' and attachment principles by a number of psychotherapies. I think these claims also reflect a lack of understanding about the developmental timeframes, family systemic conditions, and social care systemic influences that facilitate a *natural recovery* from attachment-related difficulties, without input from psychotherapists. For many children in care and adopted children, mental health recovery occurs slowly and naturally over a period of several years – if they are fortunate to have sensitive, loving and committed caregivers; if their placements are permanently maintained (even if they have a legally permanent placement); and if they do not encounter too many assaults on their felt security from social care systemic pressures. The therapeutic mechanisms contained within these developmental conditions in alternate care and adoption can largely be explained by attachment theory (Schofield & Beek, 2005). To a large extent also, many of the mental health interventions designed specifically for children in care and adopted children work towards establishing and maintaining these conditions for natural recovery – often through supporting and sustaining caregivers, and by attempting to counter harmful caregiver reactions to children's attachment difficulties.

At this chapter's end, my plea to researchers and clinicians alike is to stay mindful of the centrality of enduring, loving relationships for children's psychological development and well-being, and the role this can play in their recovery from mental ill-health – even when their difficulties appear incompatible with normal family life. With this in mind, treatment goals for children in care and adopted children should at the very least include:

- Reducing symptoms that are subjectively distressing and/or impair children's social functioning.
- Increasing children's felt security and sense of well-being.
- Strengthening children's relationships within loving, permanent families, or (if their present placement is necessarily impermanent), strengthening their capacity to form and sustain meaningful relationships with a permanent family.

Note

1 I have assumed that various study publications dating from 2000 to 2009 refer to a single RCT carried out in Oregon, reporting various analyses carried out at different stages of sample recruitment. However, the publications may instead be referring to two separate RCTs.

References

Australian Psychological Society. (2010). *Evidence-based psychological interventions in the treatment of mental disorders: A literature review (3rd Edition)*. Melbourne: Australian Psychological Society.

Barth, R. P., Crea, T., John, K., Thoburn, J., & Quinton, D. (2005). 'Beyond attachment theory and therapy: Towards sensitive and evidence-based interventions with foster and adoptive families in distress'. *Child and Family Social Work*, 10, 257–268.

Biehal, N., Dixon, J., Parry, E., Sinclair, I., Green, J., Roberts, C., (2012). *The Care Placements Evaluation (CAPE): Evaluation of Multidimensional Treatment Foster Care for Adolescents (MTFC-A)*.

Chaffin, M., Hanson, R., Saunders, B., Nichols, T., Barnett, D., Zeanah, C., (2006). 'Report of the APSAC task force on attachment therapy, Reactive Attachment Disorder, and attachment problems'. *Child Maltreatment*, 11(1), 76–89.

Chamberlain, P. (2003). 'The Oregon Multidimensional Treatment Foster Care model: Features, outcomes, and progress in dissemination'. *Cognitive and Behavioral Practice*, 10, 303–312.

Chamberlain, P., Price, J. M., Leve, L., Laurent, H., Landsverk, J., & Reid, J. (2008). 'Prevention of behavior problems for children in foster care: Outcomes and mediation effects'. *Prevention Science*, 9, 17–27.

Craven, P., & Lee, R. (2006). 'Therapeutic interventions for foster children: A systematic research synthesis'. *Research on Social Work Practice*, 16(3), 287–304.

Dallos, R., & Dallos, A. (2013). 'Using an attachment narrative approach with families where the children are looked after or adopted'. In M. Tarren-Sweeney & A. Vetere (Eds.), *Mental health services for vulnerable children and young people: Supporting children who are, or have been, in foster care*. London: Routledge.

DeJong, M. (2010). 'Some reflections on the use of psychiatric diagnosis in the looked after or "in care" child population'. *Clinical Child Psychology and Psychiatry*, 15(4), 589–599.

Dozier, M. (2003). 'Attachment-based treatment for vulnerable children'. *Attachment and Human Development*, 5(3), 253–257.

Dozier, M., Albus, K. E., Fisher, P. A., & Sepulveda, S. (2002). 'Interventions for foster parents: Implications for developmental theory'. *Development and Psychopathology*, 14, 843–860.

Dozier, M., Bick, J., & Bernard, K. (2011). 'Attachment-based treatment for young, vulnerable children'. In J. Osofsky & A. Lieberman (Eds.), *Clinical work with traumatized young children*. New York: Guilford Press.

Dozier, M., Lindheim, O., Lewis, E., Bick, J., Bernard, K., & Peloso, E. (2009). 'Effects of a foster parent training program on young children's attachment behaviors: Preliminary evidence from a randomized clinical trial'. *Child and Adolescent Social Work Journal*, 26, 321–332.

Dozier, M., Peloso, E., Lewis, E., Laurenceau, J., & Levine, S. (2008). 'Effects of an attachment-based intervention on the cortisol production of infants and toddlers in foster care'. *Development and Psychopathology*, 20, 845–859.

Dozier, M., Peloso, E., Lindheim, O., Gordon, M. K., Manni, M., Sepulveda, S., et al. (2006). 'Developing evidence-based interventions for foster children: An example of a randomized clinical trial with infants and toddlers'. *Journal of Social Issues*, 62(4), 767–785.

Fisher, P. A., Burraston, B., & Pears, K. (2005). 'The Early Intervention Foster Care program: Permanent placement outcomes from a randomized trial'. *Child Maltreatment*, 10(1), 61–71.

Fisher, P. A., Gunnar, M., Chamberlain, P., & Reid, J. (2000). 'Preventive intervention for maltreated preschool children: Impact on children's behavior, neuroendocrine activity, and foster parent functioning'. *Journal of the American Academy of Child & Adolescent Psychiatry*, 39(11), 1356.

Fisher, P. A., & Kim, H. (2007). 'Intervention effects on foster preschoolers' attachment-related behaviors from a randomized trial'. *Prevention Science*, 8, 161–170.

Fisher, P. A., Kim, H., & Pears, K. (2009). 'Effects of Multidimensional Treatment Foster Care for Preschoolers (MTFC-P) on reducing permanent placement failures among children with placement instability'. *Children and Youth Services Review*, 31, 541–546.

Fonagy, P., & Bateman, A. (2006). 'Mechanisms of change in mentalization-based treatment of BPD'. *Journal of Clinical Psychology*, 62(4), 411–430.

Fonagy, P., Target, M., Cottrell, D., Phillips, J., & Kurtz, Z. (2005). *What works for whom? A critical review of treatments for children and adolescents* (2nd ed.). New York: Guilford Press.

Howe, D. (2006). 'Developmental attachment psychotherapy with fostered and adopted children'. *Child & Adolescent Mental Health*, 11(3), 128–134.

Hughes, D. (2004). 'An attachment-based treatment for maltreated children and young people'. *Attachment and Human Development*, 6(3), 263–278.

James, S. (2011). 'What works in group care? A structured review of treatment models for group homes and residential care'. *Children and Youth Services Review*, 33(2), 308–321.

Kazdin, A. E. (2007). 'Mediators and mechanisms of change in psychotherapy research'. *Annual Review of Clinical Psychology*, 3, 1–27.

Landsverk, J., Burns, B., Stambaugh, L., & Reutz, J. (2006). *Mental health care for children and adolescents in foster care: Review of research literature*: Casey Family Programs.

——(2009). 'Psychosocial interventions for children and adolescents in foster care: Review of research literature'. *Child Welfare*, 88(1), 49–69.

Leve, L., Harold, G., Chamberlain, P., Landsverk, J., Fisher, P. A., & Vostanis, P. (2012). 'Practitioner review: Children in foster care – vulnerabilities and evidence-based interventions that promote resilience processes'. *Journal of Child Psychology & Psychiatry*, 53, 1197–1211.

MacDonald, G., & Turner, W. (2008). *Treatment foster care for improving outcomes in children and young people (Review)*: Cochrane Collaboration.

Midgley, N. (2009). 'Editorial: Improvers, adapters and rejecters – The link between "evidence-based practice" and "evidence-based practitioners"'. *Clinical Child Psychology & Psychiatry*, 14(3), 323–327.

Monck, E., Reynolds, J., & Wigfall, V. (2004). 'Using concurrent planning to establish permanency for looked after young children'. *Child & Family Social Work*, 9, 321–331.

NICE, & SCIE. (2010). *Promoting the quality of life of looked-after children and young people: Public health guidance PH28.* London: NICE / SCIE.

O'Connor, T., Matias, C., Futh, A., Tantam, G., & Scott, S. (In Press). 'Social learning theory parenting intervention promotes attachment-based caregiving in young children: Randomized clinical trial'. *Journal of Clinical Child & Adolescent Psychology*.

Price, J. M., Chamberlain, P., Landsverk, J., & Reid, J. (2009). 'KEEP foster-parent training intervention: Model description and effectiveness'. *Child and Family Social Work*, 14, 233–242.

Price, J. M., Chamberlain, P., Landsverk, J., Reid, J., Leve, L., & Laurent, H. (2008). 'Effects of a foster parent training intervention on placement changes of children in foster care'. *Child Maltreatment*, 13(1), 64–75.

Racusin, R., Maerlender, A., Sengupta, A., Isquith, P., & Straus, M. (2005). 'Psychosocial treatment of children in foster care: A review'. *Community Mental Health Journal*, 41(2), 199–221.

Royal Australian & New Zealand College of Psychiatrists. (2008). *The mental health care needs of children in out-of-home care: A report from the expert working committee of the Faculty of Child and Adolescent Psychiatry.* Melbourne: RANZCP.

Rushton, A., & Monck, E. (2009). *Enhancing adoptive parenting*. London: BAAF.

Schofield, G., & Beek, M. (2005). 'Providing a secure base: Parenting children in long-term foster family care'. *Attachment and Human Development*, 7(1), 3–25.

Tarren-Sweeney, M. (2013). 'The Assessment Checklist for Adolescents – ACA: A scale for measuring the mental health of young people in foster, kinship, residential and adoptive care'. *Children and Youth Services Review*, 35, 384–393.

——(In Press). 'An investigation of complex attachment- and trauma-related symptomatology among children in foster and kinship care'. *Child Psychiatry and Human Development*. Online first, DOI: 10.1007/s10578-013-0366-x.

Timmer, S., Urquiza, A., & Zebell, N. (2006). 'Challenging foster caregiver - maltreated child relationships: The effectiveness of parent-child interaction therapy'. *Children and Youth Services Review*, 28, 1–19.

Turner, W., MacDonald, G., & Dennis, J. (2009). *Behavioural and cognitive behavioural training interventions for assisting foster carers in the management of difficult behaviour (Review)*: Cochrane Collaboration.

Weiner, D., Schneider, A., & Lyons, J. (2009). 'Evidence-based treatments for trauma among culturally diverse foster care youth: Treatment retention and outcomes'. *Children and Youth Services Review*, 31, 1199–1205.

Part II
Recent innovations in mental health service delivery

4 Enhancing adoptive parenting
From a trial of effectiveness to translation
Alan Rushton[1]

Summary

This chapter reports on a pragmatic randomised controlled trial to evaluate two parenting programmes designed for adopters of children late placed from care. Adoptive parents, with children between 3 and 8 years who were screened to have serious behavioural problems early in the placement, participated in home-based, manualised, parenting programmes delivered by trained and supervised family social workers. The adopters who agreed to join the study were randomly allocated to one of two parenting interventions or to a 'services as usual' group. Baseline, immediate post-intervention and 6-month follow-ups were assessed using questionnaires and adopter interviews. No cases were lost to follow-up at any point and satisfaction was high with both parenting interventions. At the 6-month follow-up, outcomes for the combined intervention groups showed a significant difference (p < 0.007) in 'satisfaction with parenting' compared with the control group (Effect Size d = 0.7). Negative parenting approaches were reduced in the intervention group. However, no significant differences in child problems were found between the intervention groups and control group, adjusting for baseline scores. Costs analysis showed that a relatively modest investment in post-adoption support would be well spent in improving adopters' satisfaction with parenting in the intervention group compared to the routine service group. The chapter ends with an update on comparable adopter parenting programmes currently on offer in the UK.

Introduction

Children placed for adoption after infancy will mostly have been taken into care because of serious adversity, and most will have experienced disruptions in early relationships, and moves between carers. Not surprisingly the children have an increased risk for psycho-social difficulties. In the Maudsley Adoption and Fostering study, Quinton et al (1998) found 56% of their sample of children late placed for adoption rated over the cut-off for emotional and behavioural difficulties and no significant change in overall problem scores was evident over the first year of placement. The problems of children placed from care can challenge even experienced parents. Research has shown that the presence of conduct, overactivity and relationship problems are the ones most likely to predict poor adoption outcomes (Quinton et al, 1998; Selwyn et al, 2006). In addition to the risk of disruption, difficulties have been found to persist at an adolescent follow-up of late placements (Rushton and Dance, 2006). Clearly these children can pose a severe parenting challenge to the adopters (Rushton et al, 2003) who have often lacked an effective post-adoption support service, and for whom there is a pressing need to develop evidence-based interventions that make a positive difference to these riskier placements.

A study was therefore needed to test the effectiveness of an intervention early in the adoptive placement with samples representing the usual range of local authority adoptions rather than self-referrals to specialist adoption services. Parenting interventions were chosen in an attempt to modify the everyday home environment of the child with the expectation that the child's difficulties would reduce in time. It was hypothesised that an improvement in adoptive parenting and a reduction in the children's difficulties would be greater in the intervention groups compared with a 'service as usual' group 6 months after the intervention.

Method

Recruiting and selecting the adoptive families

Families were included in the initial recruitment stage of the study if they had a child placed for non-relative adoption between 3 and 18 months previously. All the children were between the ages of 3 years and 7 years 11 months at the time of placement and were not suffering from severe physical or learning difficulties. Children placed with relatives or with existing foster parents were excluded.

Local authorities in England with high rates of adoption were contacted and asked to identify eligible adoptive families. The help of the family's social worker was enlisted to ask the adoptive parents to complete a Strengths & Difficulties Questionnaire (SDQ) (Goodman, 2001) on each eligible child in the family. At the same time the social worker with current knowledge of the child's behaviour was also asked to complete an SDQ. The interventions were to be targeted on families whose children were exhibiting severe difficulties. When a child had a total difficulties score on either the parent's (> 13) or the social worker's (> 11) SDQ (or both), the adopters became eligible to join the study. As only one child in each family could be the focus of the interventions, the child with the highest score was selected for study.

Adopters who agreed to join the intervention study returned a signed consent form. Before the first interview the local researcher studied the child's file to collect data on the child's characteristics and history. This provided a record that was independent of the adopters' perceptions, and had the added advantage of shortening the first research interview.

The two parenting interventions

Both parenting interventions were designed to help the adopters to be in better control of the difficult behaviour and to provide the child with a consistent, responsive parenting environment. Where the adopters were a couple, both were encouraged to participate in the intervention.

The cognitive behavioural approach

The most direct influence in writing the manual for this approach has been the work of Webster-Stratton (2003). Adoptive parents are shown how to increase acceptable behaviour by using praise and rewards, to ignore unacceptable behaviour, by setting firm limits and by using 'logical consequences' and problem-solving.

The adaptation of this parenting programme was undertaken in collaboration with a clinical psychologist (Dr Helen Upright). It involves even greater emphasis on the need for adopters to conduct daily play sessions with their child and in helping them when their child rejects their praise and/ or their rewards. This intervention includes a cognitive element because parenting behaviour is influenced by how adopters come to see their child (White, McNally, & Cartwright-Hatton, 2003).

The educational approach

The 'educational' manual was designed specifically for this study with the assistance of a county adoption adviser (Mary Davidson). The aim is to improve the adopters' understanding of the meaning of the children's current behaviour and to help them to see how past and present might be connected. It addresses the constructions that the adopters place on the child's behaviour enabling them to respond appropriately, to anticipate events and thereby increase their ability to manage the behaviour.

The parent advisers for this programme were required to consult the local authority adoption files prior to meeting the adopters, in order to brief themselves on the new family and the child's history. For a more detailed account of the rationale and content of both these programmes see Rushton and Monck (2009) and Rushton et al (2010). Some of the 'service as usual' group received support, but it was far less intensive and focused than the individualised parenting advice provided in the trial.

Recruitment and training for the parent advisers

Experienced child and family social workers familiar with adoption were enlisted to act as parent advisers. They were trained to use one of the interventions and were provided with the manual and guidance on its use. Supervision was available from one of the respective practice consultants.

Randomisation and pre- and post-intervention research interviews

The first research interview took place before the family was allocated to a particular arm of the trial (Time 1, T1). Random allocation of the adoptive parents was organised independently by the Mental Health and Neuroscience Clinical Trials Unit at the Institute of Psychiatry. Permuted block randomisation was conducted to ensure that intervention group and control group numbers were evenly balanced. 'Blindness' at follow-up interviews was not possible as the adopters' involvement in the intervention or control condition was the focus of questions in the interview. The second research interview was held within two weeks of the end of the parent adviser completing the intervention, or (for the control group) about 12 weeks after the first interview (Time 2, T2). The final interview was held nine months after the first interview (Time 3, T3). All interviews with adopters were conducted in their own homes using a semi-structured format. The interviews had in common a focus on the adopters' ways of handling any problems and on the child's current behaviour and/or mood. Following the 6-month interviews adopters allocated to the control group were offered the choice of one of the parenting interventions.

Outcome measures

Child-based measures

Strengths and Difficulties Questionnaire (SDQ, Goodman, 2001) (T1, T2 & T3 to adopters). This well-established measure of children's psycho-social problems consists of 25 items relating to five scales covering emotions, behaviour, restlessness and concentration, peer relationships and prosocial behaviour (helping and caring). The first four scales are added together to provide a total difficulties score and a separately rated scale estimates the 'impact' of the difficulties. Using the SDQ to evaluate change related to intervention is regarded as an acceptable use by Goodman (see SDQinfo website).

Expression of Feelings Questionnaire (EFQ) (T1, 2, 3). This questionnaire, completed by adopters (Quinton, Rushton, Dance, & Mayes, 1998) was designed to capture the nature and progress of the relationship with the new carers by tapping the child's ability to show feelings and to seek comfort and affection appropriately. It covers distorted ways of expressing emotions as in the 'bottling up' of feelings or over-expressiveness or exhibiting affection lacking 'genuineness'. There are 50 questions employing a five-point response scale (rated 0–4); a higher score indicates better adjustment.

Post Placement Problems (PPP) (T1, 2, 3) is a nine-item adopter-completed questionnaire designed for this study and includes common problems of maltreated children when placed in a new home e.g. rejecting the new parents. The selected items are not present in the SDQ or EFQ. Each of nine items is scored 'Never', 'Sometimes', 'Often', 'Very often', and 'Always' (0–4; Maximum score 36) where a high score indicates more problematic behaviour.

Visual Analogue Scales (T3 only) tap the adopters' judgement as to how far the child has progressed in the three dimensions on which adopters have been asked detailed questions at each interview: emotional distress, misbehaviour and attachment. The adopters are asked to mark on a line whether their child's behaviour in each dimension has improved, stayed the same (centre point) or deteriorated.

Parent-based measures

The Parenting Sense of Competence Scale (PSOC) (T1, 2, 3) records a sense of satisfaction and efficacy with the parenting role (Johnston & Mash, 1989). It is based on 17 statements with six-point Likert scaling from 'Strongly agree' to 'Strongly disagree'.

Daily Hassles (T1, 2, 3) is a 20-item questionnaire designed to reflect common experiences that can pose a parenting challenge, e.g. meal time difficulties, sibling arguments (Crnic & Booth, 1991). The frequency scale records how often the events occur; the impact scale indicates the parent's subjective appraisal of how much the event affects them. There is no cut-off point, but scores above 50 on the frequency scale or above 70 on the impact scale indicate significant problems.

The Satisfaction with Parenting Advice Questionnaire is a modified version of the Parental Feedback Questionnaire (Davies & Spurr, 1998) and administered post-intervention to adopters who had received the parent adviser service.

Intervention feedback forms: Adopters and parent advisers completed feedback forms covering their responses to each session, what the adopters found more or less helpful and what the parent advisers thought about delivering the intervention.

Economic costs

The number of intervention sessions that the families received was recorded and used to estimate the total cost of the interventions. Other service use was measured using an adapted version of the Client Service Receipt Inventory (Beecham and Knapp, 2001). Services were retrospectively recorded for the period between placement and baseline assessment, and then for the follow-up periods. Services included contacts with social work and health, and educational input. Unit costs, obtained from a recognised source

66 Alan Rushton

(Curtis, 2007), were attached to the service use data in order to generate total service costs.

Statistical analysis

Initial power calculations indicated that in order to detect a difference in outcome with 80% power using a significance level of $p < 0.05$, 27 cases would be needed in each group. In the event, due to numerous recruitment obstacles, 37 families entered the trial out of the 178 screened (see Figure 4.1 for flow chart). Due to this relatively small sample size the statistical analysis was mainly conducted by combining the cases in the two intervention groups and comparing their outcomes with the 'service as usual' cases.

The effectiveness of the parenting interventions was assessed at post intervention and at the 6-month follow-up by analysis of variance, controlling for baseline values. Effect sizes were estimated using Cohen's D (Cohen, 1988). Cost-differences were assessed using bootstrapped regression models with the group identifier (intervention or service as usual) entered as a single

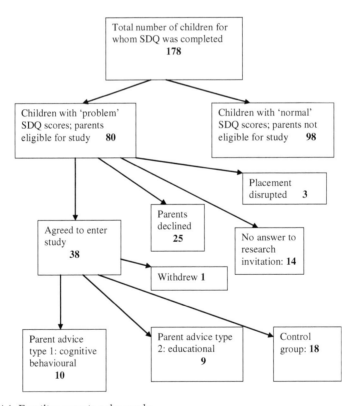

Figure 4.1 Families entering the study

independent variable. Bootstrapping was used because of the likely non-normal distribution of the regression residuals.

Results

Of 80 families screened as eligible, 37 entered the trial. The adoptive placements were made between 2004 and 2006 and no placement disruptions occurred in the sample during the research period. The children were mostly placed with couples, of which three were same sex partners; nine children lived with single adoptive parents. All but one of the families completed the full ten parenting advice sessions and all families completed the follow-up research interviews.

For the total sample entering the trial, the average age of the index child at the adoptive placement was 5½ years (67 months, sd = 18 months, range = 36–102 months) and by the time of the first research interview the children had been placed for an average of 12 months (range = 5–18 months). A simple count of pre-placement major adversities (e.g. parental abuse) noted on the files showed a mean of seven adversities (range = 2–13). Table 4.1 gives a comparison of the intervention groups and control group in terms of the child's characteristics and pre-placement history. The randomised groups were well balanced. Tables 4.2 and 4.3 give the outcome data comparing interventions with controls.

Strengths and Difficulties Questionnaire completed by adopters

In terms of the whole sample, regardless of group allocation, mean SDQ scores remained well above the cut-off 6 months after the intervention. The mean level of total difficulties reduced very little for the whole group (Time 1: 19.78, sd 6.0; Time 2: 18.65, sd 6.3; Time 3: 17.86, sd 6.1). Linear regression analysis was conducted (at T2 with T1 as a covariate, and at T3 with T1 as covariate) to compare the combined intervention group with the control group. No significant differences were found between baseline and post-intervention SDQ scores, and baseline and six-month post-intervention follow-up scores, nor between the interventions groups and the control group. In addition, no significant differences were found on any of the problem sub-scales, pro-social or SDQ impact scores at T2 or T3.

Expression of Feelings Questionnaire

EFQ total scores were higher (i.e. more positive) at all time points for the intervention group and the general pattern showed a rise for the intervention group scores and little change for the controls, but differences were not significant at T2 and T3 when controlling for the baseline scores.

68 Alan Rushton

Table 4.1 Characteristics of children randomised to intervention and control groups

	Intervention group (n = 19)	Control group (n = 18)
Child		
Sex (% girls)	53	55
Ethnicity – (% white)	84	88
Mean age at placement in months (SD)	68 (19)	65 (17)
Age at first admission to care in months (SD)	37 (14)	27 (17)
Mean no. of changes of placement (SD)	6 (2.9)	6 (3.7)
SDQ score at baseline Mean (SD)	18 (4.1)	20 (7.3)
Reason for first admission to care	percent	percent
Neglect	89	89
Sexual abuse	21	22
Physical abuse	58	44
Emotional abuse	57	33
Carer's mental illness	47	39
Carer's addiction	42	72
Concern about sibs	56	43
Schedule 1 offender in household	16	22
Domestic violence	63	55
Other adversities		
Prematurity	16	22
Perinatal problems	22	11
Mother's addiction during pregnancy	6	33
Broken attachments	84	44
Parental conflict	47	55
Parental withdrawal from child	36	39
Severe economic deprivation	52	61
Parenting experiences		
Any positive parenting (physical)	21	22
Any positive parenting (psychosocial)	21	17
Negative parenting in first 2 years	69	78
Any good parenting >2 years (physical)	63	67
Any good parenting >2 years (psychosocial)	58	61
Child's major health problem	16	33
Total no. of adversities on file		
Mean and SD	8.21 (3.0)	7.22 (2.4)

Post Placement Problems Questionnaire

The control group had higher mean problem scores than the intervention group at T2 and T3 but not significantly so when controlling for baseline scores.

Parenting Sense of Competence scales

In the combined intervention groups the Satisfaction with parenting score improved (34 at T1, to 37 at T2 and 39, at T3) whereas for the controls

Table 4.2 Outcomes at immediate post-intervention (Time 2)

Outcome measures at T2	Mean differences at T2 and 95% CI	Adjusted mean differences (B) and 95% CI	Effect size Cohen's d	P value adjusted	In favour of...
SDQ total difficulties T2	−0.18 −4.4 to 4.0	−2.13 −5.72 to 1.45	0.35	p= 0.23	Control Group
Expression of Feelings Questionnaire total scores	−14.7 −29.9 to 0.49	−10.4 −23.4 to 2.5	0.49	p=0.11	Intervention groups
Post-placement problems	1.23 −2.6 to 5.1	0.08 −3.25 to 3.0	0.01	p= 0.95	Intervention groups
Parenting Sense of Competence: Satisfaction with parenting	−1.05 −5.84 to 3.73	−2.09 −5.94 to 1.75	0.31	p= 0.27	Intervention groups
Parenting efficacy	−2.03 −6.49 to 2.41	−1.3 −4.93 to 2.32	0.20	p= 0.46	Intervention groups
Daily hassles: Frequency	4.3 −1.67 to 10.4	1.81 −2.55 to 6.19	0.25	p= 0.4	Intervention groups
Daily hassles: Intensity	7.04 − 2.2 to 16.03	7.01 −1.16 to 15.19	0.53	p= 0.09	Intervention groups

All differences calculated as Control minus Intervention scores
Adjusted mean differences at T2 (B) controlling for T1 (linear regression)
Cohen's d calculated on the basis of adjusted mean differences

Table 4.3 Outcomes at six months post intervention (Time 3)

Outcome measures at T3	Mean differences at T3 and 95% CI	Adjusted mean differences (B) and 95% CI	Effect size Cohen's d	P value adjusted	In favour of…
Parents' SDQ total difficulties T3	1.04 −3.15 to 5.24	−0.79= −4.45 to 2.85	0.13	p= 0.66	Control Group
Expression of Feelings Questionnaire total score	−11.2 −26.0 to 3.5	−6.18 −17.2 to 4.8	0.29	p= 0.26	Intervention groups
Post-placement problems	−3.22 −8.8 to 2.37	−0.91 −2.17 to 3.99	0.21	p= 0.55	Intervention groups
Parenting sense of competence: Satisfaction with parenting	−3.67 −8.4 to 1.1	4.9 −8.4 to −1.4	0.7	p= 0.007	Intervention groups
Parenting efficacy	−3.41 −7.92 to 1.64	−2.26 −5.86 to 1.33	0.34	p = 0.21	Intervention groups
Daily hassles: Frequency	−0.97 −5.5 to 7.4	−0.91 −5.4 to 3.5	0.13	p= 0.68	Control Group
Daily hassles: Intensity	1.29 −6.4 to 6.4	1.78 −4.7 to 8.34	0.13	p= 0.58	Intervention groups

Adjusted mean differences at T3 (B) controlling for T1 (linear regression) the Satisfaction score stayed fairly constant (T1 - 37, T2 - 36, T3 - 35). At the 6-month follow-up, a highly significant difference (p<0.007, 95% CI – 8.4 to –1.4) and large Effect Size (d = 0.7) was found in favour of the combined intervention group. The Efficacy score on PSOC did not show a significant difference as both scores rose over time.

Daily Hassles

Adjusted mean differences for the combined intervention group and the control group were mostly not significant on either the Frequency or the Intensity scales. Although scores were higher on the intensity scale for the control group at T2 (p < 0.09), indicating more problems, at T3 differences were not significant.

Adopters' satisfaction with the parenting interventions

The summary scores on the Satisfaction with Parental Advice Questionnaire indicated high satisfaction levels; there were no differences between the two intervention groups.

Analogue Scales

The adopters generally recorded their children as having made some progress: only 22% recorded that their child had deteriorated in the field of emotional distress; 19% in behaviour; and 5% in attachment. However, there were no differences between the intervention groups and the control group on the extent and direction of change.

Cost-effectiveness analysis

The costs of services used by participants before baseline and at each follow-up interview were measured. The costs during the period up to post-treatment follow-up were £1528 higher for the intervention group than the routine care group – a difference that was not statistically significant. Costs over the entire follow-up period were £1652 higher for the intervention groups. This was not significant due to the high level of variation in the cost. The cost-effectiveness analysis revealed that in terms of the SDQ, routine care was dominant (better outcomes and lower costs). However, regarding parent satisfaction the intervention was more effective. Costs of £731 would be incurred to achieve a point improvement in satisfaction compared to routine care by the end of treatment.

For a relatively modest investment in post-adoption support, evidence can now be cited from this study to show that this money would be well spent in enhancing parenting.

(Full details of the economic analysis are published elsewhere (Sharac et al, 2011).)

The qualitative findings

Adopters' reports on handling the difficulties

Significantly more adopters said they handled emotional difficulties differently at T2 compared with T1 ($\chi 2$ 7.9, df 1, p < 0.005) and at T3 compared with T2 ($\chi 2$ 4.5, df 1, p < 0.03). Very little difference was apparent in the way that adopters from the two groups dealt with misbehaviour to begin with, but at T2 the control group used significantly more 'threats' ($\chi 2 = 5.9$, df 1, p < 0.01). At T3, the controls were no longer using more threats, but were still 'telling off' ($\chi 2$ 4.5, df 1, p < 0.03) and 'shouting' ($\chi 2 = 4.9$, df 1, p < 0.02) significantly more than the intervention group. The frequency of relationship problems was compared across the interventions and controls and at the three time points. None showed a significant difference except 'indiscriminate relationships' at T3 which was less frequent in the intervention groups with the difference approaching significance ($\chi 2$ 2.9, df = 1, p < 0.08).

Differences between the interventions

The trial design provided the opportunity to compare and contrast the two interventions - at least via the qualitative data, although the small numbers limited the statistical comparison. Both interventions were highly valued but with some differences in the adopters' responses. The adopters in the behavioural group said they were helped to carry through the behavioural advice consistently and persistently while the education group adopters valued the opportunity to stand back and reach a better understanding of the problems with the assistance of a knowledgeable and experienced practitioner.

Adopter and adviser feedback forms

The adopters almost universally responded positively to the interventions. The weekly advice sessions were in most cases reported to be much more intensive than the adoption support given before. One aspect of the advice service that stood out was the benefit of working through problems with the same trusted adviser, and contrasted with the generalised parenting advice most families had received before placement. The advisers strongly supported aspects of the manuals devoted to the benefits of relaxed time for play, but found the manuals less helpful in relation to aggressive and dangerous behaviour.

Reflections on the research findings and on the challenges of conducting a 'real world' randomised controlled trial

This study has examined the effectiveness of parenting advice provided to adopters facing serious challenges from their children's behaviour during the first 18 months of placement. On the basis of the parenting measure and of feedback from the adopters, they were shown to have greater capacity for change than the children. Significant differences were found between the groups of adopters at 6 months' follow-up on the Parenting Sense of Competence Scale indicating that satisfaction in parenting their child rose after receiving advice sessions, while the satisfaction level of the control group fell slightly. For the intervention group, raised satisfaction might provide a stronger basis for dealing with future problems. The adopters frequently drew attention to one particular advantage of the individualised parent advice sessions: they were able to talk exclusively about the problems presented by the index child.

However, no significant differences were apparent between the intervention group and the control group regarding a reduction in the children's psycho-social problems. The question has to be posed as to why the high level of problems persisted regardless of the passage of time and the interventions. A number of explanations may be relevant, especially the enduring effects of extremely adverse events and circumstances before coming into care and multiple changes of placement. Other factors may have been present but not captured in this trial like pre-natal exposure to toxins and peri-natal hazards. Both genetic vulnerability and greater susceptibility to adversity may mean that these children are less responsive to any therapeutic aspects of the new adoptive environment. The children were selected into the trial because they had a high level of problems. It might therefore seem over-optimistic to expect these difficulties to reduce substantially in a relatively short time. Perhaps the beneficial influence of a longer period of stable, positive family life would be necessary to see significant change and even then some effects of earlier maltreatment might not readily be remedied. As children were only selected for the trial when having severe problems, it is important that the results of the trial are not generalised to all late adoptive placements.

Design and measurement issues

Sample size and representativeness

Although an RCT design helps potentially to gain more control over the many variables pertinent to an intervention, in a 'real-world' trial it is not always easy to achieve adequate sample size and representativeness. Several factors appear to have made an impact on the lower than anticipated recruitment figures. For instance, the number of adopters with children screened for serious difficulties who declined to join the study was considerably higher than expected. Only some of the parents who did not join gave their reasons, so one can only speculate on what determined entrance to the trial. But it is of interest to question why adopters with children exhibiting severe difficulties by their own account, decline a free, home-delivered, adopter tailored service.

The shortfall in intended recruitment inevitably limits the strength of the study's conclusions. The planned sample size proved impossible to achieve even when the number of participating authorities was increased and the time scale extended. Ethical requirements meant adopters could not be approached directly but had to use their social workers as intermediaries. The strictest assessment would be that the study does not have enough power to test the hypothesis, leading to the blunt conclusion that the outcome data cannot be used to support implications for effective practice. By contrast it could be argued that the relatively small sample size is somewhat compensated for by the fact that the adopters attended virtually all sessions of the ten week programme and nearly complete data were gathered on all cases and at all follow-up points. Analysis with minimal missing data resulted in fewer of the usual frustrations, and reduced the potential for bias, an equally important issue alongside sample size and power.

Outcome measures and sensitivity to change

A major issue in RCT design is the choice of measure to be used to record change. It was important to use at least one standard instrument to measure child outcome because of its proven reliability and the existence of known population norms. Most intervention studies choose from the commonly used child mental health measures although they were not necessarily designed as change measures. However, there may also be a problem of content. The questionnaire used in this study – the SDQ – largely assesses anti-social behaviour and depressed mood. In adoptive placements these issues are of high importance to the parents but so also is attachment behaviour that is weak or inappropriate. The SDQ is not designed to tap these problems. Other issues that emerged in the interviews were the highly controlling behaviour of some children, extreme physical aggression and emotional dysregulation. Outcome measures must represent in ex-care adopted children the broad spectrum of difficulties and the importance of small but meaningful changes. The SDQ ratings (not true, somewhat true, or certainly true) do not allow for the fine tuning that may make parents feel that progress is being made. An example might relate to tantrums: perhaps initially occurring two or three times a day, but reducing to perhaps six times a week would still be recorded as 'certainly true', while parents might feel that the child was definitely 'better'.

Implementing the Enhanced Adoptive Parenting (EAP) RCT findings

As both parenting manuals were equally appreciated, as neither showed superior results and as adopters generally wanted both 'understanding' and 'strategies', there was a strong case for combining the manuals into a single document after the trial. The next stage of the work was therefore to take account of the feedback from the adopters and the parent advisors and to incorporate changes into a Mark 11, 10 session version of the manual. Accordingly the following changes were made:

- More information was given of the origins and nature of attachment difficulties
- Coverage was increased on aggression and dangerous behaviour by the child
- More attention was paid to the advice adopters found difficult to follow, e.g. ignoring difficult behaviour
- An 'optional extras' section was added to cover those less frequent problems that were nevertheless presenting a challenge for some families. These included wetting and soiling, sexualised behaviour, sibling and peer relationships, fears and anxieties and eating and sleeping problems.

This improved version was then piloted on six new adoptive parents to check on its acceptability and whether it was working satisfactorily. The presentation of the manual was improved for publication and a CD-ROM included which contained the handouts so that they could be easily printed off by parent advisers. It was written into the guidance that when manuals are used in agency settings this should follow careful screening and assessment of families' existing skills and knowledge to decide if this parenting programme is indeed the correct focus of intervention and whether the adopters are likely to be receptive to the programme.

Since publication of the EAP manual (Rushton and Upright, 2012) the Post Adoption Centre (PAC) in London has been involved in the revision, piloting and dissemination of the programme. The PAC is a registered charity providing pre- and post-adoption services. It is now training parent advisers to use the manual and is delivering the 10-week programme to adoptive parents. Routine before and after measures of child problems and parenting change are being collected. These are small beginnings, but local authority adoption teams have shown an interest in purchasing the manual and the training programme and increasingly want to know about the evidence base for an intervention.

It is a frequent criticism of RCT findings that they only apply when the narrow conditions under which the trial was constructed are replicated. Effects may well vary if the recipients or methods used are not faithful to the original trial or are delivered by less skilled staff. Carefully negotiated partnerships between researchers and practitioners are necessary for effective translation of an evidence-based programme.

Current UK adopter parenting programmes

Obvious common aims of adopter parenting programmes are the reduction of placement disruption rates, improvement in the quality of adoptive family life and lessening the current and possible longer-term mental health problems in the children. However, such programmes can be delivered in a variety of ways. They may differ in length, structure, frequency and timing – all of which may affect accessibility, attendance and drop-out rates. They vary in who provides the parenting advice and the training system. Programmes may be individual or group-based, home-based or agency-based, with or without a published manual or handbook. They give different levels of attention to the elements of parent education, understanding, skills and self-care. Theoretical orientations span the usual divisions in developmental psychology from the social learning approach to the psychoanalytic. Some programmes promote practical everyday help to adopters in managing difficult behaviour. Adaptations of the Webster-Stratton approach have been tailored for group-based sessions with adopters (see Henderson and Sargent, 2005). Others are concerned with aspects like the adopters' emotional responses, the quality of the parent–child relationship, self-reflection and the adopters' own history of being parented. The chapter will conclude with a brief review of developments and evaluations of three selected adoptive parenting programmes currently on offer in the UK.

It's a piece of cake? is an example of a group-based, six-module programme developed to meet the demands of adopters with challenging children. Accredited Adoption UK trainers who are adopters themselves provide the service. The distinguishing features of the programme include developing parenting skills, confidence building, affirmation of the adopters' own parenting methods, self-care and understanding of attachment issues. Participants are linked to a support group. Adoption UK commissioned an evaluation from the Hadley Centre for Adoption and Foster Care Studies at the University of Bristol and the Evaluation Trust (Selwyn, del Tufo & Frazer, 2009). This appears to be the UK study that most closely resembles the EAP evaluation. The programme was prospectively evaluated and compared adopters attending and not attending it. Pre- and post-training data were assessed using the well-known Strengths and Difficulties Questionnaire (SDQ) and the Expression of Feelings in Relationships Questionnaire (EFR) which was used to capture children's styles of relating to their carers. The children's scores were not found to change significantly over time nor between the experimental and control groups. However parenting style in the experimental group exhibited better understanding of the child, a wider repertoire of parenting responses, a growth in confidence and more enjoyment in playing with their children. The limitations of the evaluation, as acknowledged by the authors, were that the lack of random allocation meant that important

Enhancing adoptive parenting 77

differences between the experimental and control groups could have contributed to the outcomes and the study was unable to collect longer term post-intervention data.

'After Adoption' has developed an adopters' parenting programme called *SafeBase*. This is delivered by qualified social workers with a focus of interest on attachment theory, child development and the impact of trauma and loss. After initial observation and feedback on family interactions, four days of training are designed to give adopters advice on building relationships with their children. Theraplay sessions are included in the training to help adopters to change their child's negative behaviour and to promote attachment (Booth & Lindaman, 2000). Access is given to support groups and on line forums. The agency is keen to secure funding for an external evaluation.

The *ADOPT programme* is based on the principles of a group intervention devised originally for foster carers: the KEEP model (Keeping Foster Parents Trained and Supported). KEEP originated in the Oregon Social Learning Centre and aims to improve outcomes for children with behavioural and emotional problems by enhancing caregiver understanding and skills in managing difficult behaviour (Fisher et al, 2005). Phil Fisher is collaborating with Rosemarie Roberts (South London & Maudsley NHS trust) to tailor a programme specifically for use with adopters in the UK context. In response to demand from local authorities in England, the Department for Education has commissioned them to develop the curriculum and pilot the intervention. ADOPT is being designed as a preventative programme to be offered immediately post placement or within the first two years. Like the EAP programme, it encourages the use of positive reinforcement and the setting of clear and consistent limits. It includes role-plays and videotaped recordings and home practice assignments following group-based learning and aims to integrate social learning theory, neuroscience and attachment theory into the curriculum. At the time of writing, the team has no immediate plans for an effectiveness trial.

Three programmes have been cited above and there may well be others in development. However, if parenting manuals and internal audits are not in the public domain it is hard to see how knowledge of 'what works' can accumulate. Many adoption support agencies and local authority adoption units should, and do, assess the outcomes of their work as a matter of routine auditing and any well-conducted evaluations deserve to be peer reviewed and open to scrutiny.

Evaluating adoptive parenting programmes

The evaluations so far conducted have thrown up important questions. For example, the aspects of parenting that are being targeted need to be distinguished. There are many candidates: changes in parenting style, attitude and receptiveness; reduced negative attribution of the child's behaviour; self-exploration of the adopter's feelings towards the child; increased understanding of psychological development; greater emotional responsiveness and sensitivity, reduced stress levels and more harmonious couple relationships (where applicable). How do the programmes address this variety of targets?

Similarly many targets exist for positive change in the children. Mostly the aim is reduction in behavioural and relationship problems, but more specific aspects are being explored like emotion regulation, improved executive function and greater self-control. Strategies for achieving some of these aims, especially the promotion of greater attachment, have been much contested (see for example Allen, 2011) and despite advocacy for some newer therapeutic interventions, evidence of effectiveness is often lacking specifically in the adoption context.

Many questions remain. What are the pathways linking parenting change to child improvement? Which aspects of parenting change affect which child problems? If some maltreated children have problems across all domains, which of these are best to target and in what sequence? Which child problems can and cannot be significantly influenced by changes in parenting?

The three programmes discussed above have been concerned with interventions solely targeted on the adoptive parents. This might be broadened to include the extended family, peers and friends. Some have argued that behaviourally oriented parenting skills models are limited in not addressing core adopter/child relationship quality and strong interest has emerged in interventions that focus on promoting more positive relationships by including the child jointly in the intervention, for example Dyadic Developmental Psychotherapy (Becker-Weidman & Hughes 2008). Attunement of the adopters' and the child's attachment style may be a focus of intervention. However, a counter argument is that achieving a reduction in behavioural problems should be prioritised because this will lead to a more relaxed, less conflicted interactions from which a more mutually satisfying parent/child relationship will develop.

The example of multi-model programmes for adoptive families presents a major challenge for evaluation. This is especially so if the additional intervention is a new development which is yet to be subject to a trial. Theraplay, for example, is widely used in the field and viewed as beneficial by practitioners but still awaits a rigorous evaluation of effectiveness in the context of adoption. (One small randomised trial with birth families showed a reduction in children's internalising problems, Siu, 2009.) A package of interventions may be proposed as the best approach for a family, but an attempt to evaluate such combined inputs may be unable to distinguish the unique contribution of each element. A simpler research design may be possible whereby a 'parenting programme only' is compared with the identical programme delivered with an intervention including the child. This could potentially identify the contribution, beneficial or otherwise, of the added element.

The evaluation of foster care programmes

The number of evaluations of parenting programmes for birth parents is increasing (Scott, 2008) and more recently those for foster care training, but specific adoption intervention evaluations lag a long way behind. In the absence of many adoption-based intervention trials, it is worth learning from the evaluation of foster care programmes. The aims of such placements will be different, but the children, in having pre-placement histories of maltreatment, are likely to have similar behavioural, neurobiological and relationship problems and challenges to their carers. Randomised controlled trials of foster care interventions, more numerous in the US, have shown better outcomes for experimental over control groups on a range of measures, albeit with moderate effect sizes e.g. Multidimensional Treatment Foster Care for Preschoolers (Fisher and Kim, 2007); Attachment and Biobehavioural Catch-up (ABC) (Dozier et al, 2008); Keeping Foster Parents Trained and Supported (KEEP) (Chamberlain et al, 2008). Evidence of beneficial adoptive parenting programmes needs to see a similar increase. Any studies which are developing better measures of parenting change and more sensitive indicators of improvement in the children, especially in growth of attachment, will assist in the field of adoption research.

Rating the evidence base

Commissioners and practitioners need to be more aware of the hierarchy of persuasive evidence of effectiveness. Clearinghouse systems are being established to provide critical evaluations of intervention programmes. Top rating should be awarded to an intervention that has been subject to one RCT, and preferably more than one, in different agency settings and locations, and by independent research teams. The intervention should be theoretically justified, have a clear description of the method of intervention (a published manual), appropriate and reliable 'before and after' measures of outcome, sufficient statistical power to detect a positive change (i.e. in child and parenting measures) and follow-ups to test whether the effect is sustained beyond the intervention. The evidence should have been examined through a peer review system and published in a reputable journal. Clearly these are the most exacting standards and very few adopter parenting programmes meet all these criteria.

A middle-rated group could be labelled as promising evidence through the use of some form of before and after test and a comparison group with equalised characteristics so that effects can justifiably be attributed to the intervention. A lower rating would apply to evidence based on the opinions of services users only. This, of course, is crucial information to gather, especially to test whether the intervention has been acceptable and relevant to the adopters. It can also be informative on which aspects of a programme were thought to be most helpful or were hardest to implement. However, as most programmes report high rates of satisfaction, this may offer little help in distinguishing between them. At the bottom of the table would be programmes that have no evidence of improved outcomes, or worse, have resulted in negative changes for the parents or the child or are judged to be unethical or harmful.

Conclusions

Studies are accumulating evidence that programmes can enhance adopter parenting styles and understanding, reduce tension and increase satisfaction with parenting. These are important findings as they show that adopters do generally have the flexibility and capacity to make changes. It is reasonable to suppose that this improved parenting environment will have a beneficial effect on the child's psycho-social problems. But evidence is less forthcoming for modifying severe problems in maltreated children in the early part of an adoptive placement – at least in the short term.

Funding for further well-planned RCTs would be ideal as they produce the severest test of effectiveness, but given the complexity of setting them up and the comparatively high research costs involved, it would be surprising to see many being conducted, at least in the UK in the near future. This leaves another possibility: that is that adoption support agencies could combine their efforts in order to compare outcomes across programmes. This would increase the total number of cases in an evaluation, common measures could be employed and this could eventually produce useful information on which aspects of which programmes have what magnitude of effect.

Note

1 This study was funded initially by the UK Department of Health and the Nuffield Foundation and later by the Sir Halley Stewart Trust. Thanks go to my research colleagues: Elizabeth Monck, Morven Leese, Paul McCrone and Jessica Sharac and to Helen Upright and Mary Davidson for helping to write the parenting manuals. The study was approved by the Joint South London and Maudsley /Institute of Psychiatry Research Ethics Committee and registered as International Standard Randomised Controlled Trial Number: ISRCTN04448012.

References

Allen, B. (2011). 'The use and abuse of attachment theory in clinical practice with maltreated children, part II: Treatment'. *Trauma Violence Abuse*, *12*(1), 13–22.
Beecham, J., & Knapp, M. (2001). 'Costing psychiatric interventions'. In G. Thornicroft (Ed) *Measuring mental health needs*. London: Gaskell.

Booth, P., & Lindaman, S. (2000). 'Theraplay for enhancing attachment in adopted children'. In H. G. Kaduson, & C. E. Schaefer (Eds.) *Short-term play therapy for children* (pp. 194–227). New York, NY: Guilford Press.

Becker-Weidman, A., & Hughes, D. (2008). 'Dyadic Developmental Psychotherapy: An evidence-based treatment for children with complex trauma and disorders of attachment'. *Child and Family Social Work*, 13, 329–337.

Chamberlain, P., Price, J., Leve, L. D., Laurent, H., Landsverk, J., & Reid, J. B. (2008). 'Prevention of behavior problems for children in foster care: Outcomes and mediation effects'. *Prevention Science*, 9(1), 17–27.

Cohen, J. (1988). *Statistical power analysis for the behavioural sciences*. Hillsdale, NJ: Erlbaum.

Crnic, K. A., & Booth, C. L. (1991). 'Mothers' and fathers' perceptions of daily hassles of parenting across early childhood'. *Journal of Marriage and the Family*, 53, 1043–1050.

Curtis, L. (2007). *Unit Costs of health and social care*. Personal Social Services Research Unit, University of Kent.

Davies, H., & Spurr, P. (1998). 'Parent counselling; An evaluation of a community child mental health service'. *Journal of Child Psychology and Psychiatry*, 39, 365–376.

Dozier, M., Peloso, E., Lewis, E., Laurenceau, J., & Levine, S. (2008). 'Effects of an attachment-based intervention on the cortisol production of infants and toddlers in foster care'. *Development and Psychopathology*, 20, 845–859.

Fisher, P. A., Burraston, B., & Pears, K. (2005). 'The Early Intervention Foster Care Program: Permanent placement outcomes from a randomised trial'. *Child Maltreatment*, 10, 61–71.

Fisher, P. A., & Kim, H. K. (2007). 'Intervention effects on foster preschoolers' attachment-related behaviors from a randomised trial'. *Prevention Science*, 8, 161–170.

Goodman, R. (2001). 'Psychometric properties of the Strengths and Difficulties Questionnaire (SDQ)'. *Journal of the American Academy of Child and Adolescent Psychiatry*, 40, 1337–1345.

Henderson, K., & Sargent, N. (2005). 'Developing the Incredible years Webster-Stratton parenting skills programme for use with adoptive families'. *Adoption & Fostering*, 29(4), 34–44.

Johnston, C., & Mash, E. (1989). 'A measure of parenting satisfaction and efficacy'. *Journal of Clinical Child Psychology*, 18(2), 167–175.

Quinton, D., Rushton, A., Dance, C., & Mayes, D. (1998). *Joining new families: a study of adoption and fostering in middle childhood*. Chichester: Wiley & Sons.

Rushton, A., Mayes., Dance, C., & Quinton, D. (2003). 'Parenting late placed children: The development of new relationships and the challenge of behavioural problems'. *Clinical Child Psychology and Psychiatry*, 8, 389–400.

Rushton, A., & Dance, C. (2006). 'The adoption of children from public care: a prospective study of outcome in adolescence'. *Journal of the American Academy of Child and Adolescent Psychiatry*, 45(7), 877–883.

Rushton, A., Monck, E., Leese, M., McCrone, P., & Sharac, J. (2010). 'Enhancing adoptive parenting: a randomised controlled trial'. *Clinical Child Psychology and Psychiatry*, 15(4), 529–542.

Rushton, A., & Monck, E. (2009). *Enhancing adoptive parenting: a test of effectiveness*. London: BAAF.

Rushton, A., & Upright, H. (2012). *Enhancing adoptive parenting: a parenting programme for use with new adopters of challenging children*. London: BAAF.

Scott, S. (2008). 'Parenting programmes'. In: Rutter, M., Bishop, D., Pine, D., Scott, S., Stevenson, J., Taylor, E., & Thapar, A. (Eds.) *Rutter's child and adolescent psychiatry* (5th edition). Oxford: Blackwell.

Selwyn, J., Sturgess, W., Quinton, D., & Baxter, C. (2006). *Costs and outcomes of non-infant adoptions.* London: BAAF.

Selwyn, J., del Tufo, S., & Frazer, L. (2009). It's a Piece of Cake? An evaluation of an adopter training programme. *Adoption and Fostering, 33,* 30–43.

Sharac J., McCrone P., Rushton A., & Monck E. (2011). 'Enhancing adoptive parenting: cost effectiveness analysis'. *Child and Adolescent Mental Health, 16*(2), 110–115.

Siu, A. F. Y. (2009). 'Theraplay in the Chinese world: an intervention program for Hong Kong children with internalizing problems'. *International Journal of Play Therapy, 18,* 1–12.

Webster-Stratton, C. (2003). *The incredible years: A trouble shooting guide for parents of children aged 3-8.* Toronto, ON: The Umbrella Press.

White, C., McNally, D., & Cartwright-Hatton, S. (2003). 'Cognitively enhanced parent training'. *Behavioural and Cognitive Psychotherapy, 31,* 99–102.

5 The 'Spirit of New Orleans'[1]

Translating a model of intervention with maltreated children and their families for the Glasgow context

Helen Minnis, Graham Bryce, Louise Phin and Philip Wilson

Summary

Children in care have higher rates of mental health problems than the general population and placement instability contributes to this. Children are both most vulnerable to the effects of poor quality care and most responsive to treatment in the early weeks and months of life yet, in the UK, permanency decisions are generally not in place until around the age of four. We aimed to understand the components of an innovative system for assessing and intervening with maltreated children and their families developed in New Orleans and to consider how it might be implemented in Glasgow, UK. During and after a visit to New Orleans by a team of Glasgow practitioners, eight key interviews and meetings with New Orleans and Glasgow staff were audio-recorded. Qualitative analysis of verbatim transcripts identified key themes. Themes highlighted shared aspects of the context and attitudes of the two teams, identified gaps in the Glasgow service and steps that would be needed to implement a version of the New Orleans model in Glasgow. Our discussions with the New Orleans team have highlighted concrete steps we can take, in Glasgow, to make better decision-making for vulnerable children a reality.

Introduction

The well-being of children who experience maltreatment in their own family comes dramatically to public attention when there is a death. The recent UK cases of 'Baby P' (Healthcare Commission, 2009) and Brandon Muir (The Highland Council, 2009) illustrate graphically the risks which some children face as well as the challenges for public agencies in assessing those risks and in deciding how to respond. In this chapter we consider a particular aspect of this problem as we focus on working with young maltreated children who have been removed from the care of their parent(s) for their own safety. The context for our discussion is a collaborative project between teams in Glasgow and New Orleans who work with children in this situation. Such work, of necessity, has several objectives but there is an over-arching aim of promoting the wellbeing of the individual children. Mental health is central to that project and our discussion proceeds by considering what is known about the mental health of children in care and how the setting in which they grow up may influence that. The project is a key element of a comprehensive framework for supporting parenting in Glasgow (Wilson, Bryce, Puckering, & Minnis, 2008).

Children's mental health and care setting

The evidence about the mental health of children who are maltreated comes from the research literature and clinical reports. Several robust epidemiological studies in the UK have now confirmed that the prevalence of mental health difficulties amongst this population is significantly higher than that of their peers who were not looked after (Dimigen et al., 1999; McCann, James, Wilson, & Dunn, 1996; Meltzer, Gatward, Corbin, Goodman, & Ford, 2003), whether children were placed in family foster care, kinship (extended family) care or residential care. The mental health problems of looked after and accommodated children can be complex: it is common for children to have problems in more than one domain and, in addition, some problems (such as attachment disorder) are still challenging to assess and treat (Meltzer et al., 2003; O'Connor & Zeanah, 2003). Problems are also likely to be of complex aetiology: although genetic factors have an important part to play, even in disorders thought to be specifically associated with maltreatment (Minnis et al., 2007), one crucial aspect of the environment which can be modified is the care setting in which the child is reared.

Thankfully, the UK no longer looks after children in large institutions, but in the days when this was still common, Tizard and colleagues showed that children who returned to family care or were adopted did significantly better in their social and emotional development than children who remained in large institutions (Hodges & Tizard, 1989a; Hodges & Tizard, 1989b). The UK 2003 Office for National Statistics (ONS) survey of the mental health of children looked after by local authorities showed that rates of mental health difficulty were higher for children living in residential care than for children living in foster care (Meltzer et al, 2003). In addition, the UK has a system whereby children whose safety and well-being is of particular concern to services, but for whom there is no clear evidence of maltreatment, can be 'looked after at home' with their birth families. The ONS survey was particularly important in drawing attention to the fact that the mental health of these children is as poor, as a group, as those who are looked after in foster or residential care (Meltzer et al., 2003). The care setting in which children are reared is therefore crucial, and decisions about what kind of placement is right for a maltreated child is likely to have profound implications for that child's life course. However, several enquiries into deaths of maltreated children have demonstrated the challenges in making good decisions: getting good developmental information about children whose families are in chaos; integrating the information from different services and making sense of the way information emerges over time (Healthcare Commission, 2009; The Highland Council, 2009).

For the purposes of illustrating the importance of the decision-making process, we have developed a short account of what happens to children from Glasgow who come into the foster care for the first time before they reach the age of five:

- One-third of under-5s who come into their first episode of care remain permanently in alternative care. Of these, one in three is adopted, while two in three stay in foster care on a long-term basis.
- Two out of three under-5s who come into their first episode of care return to the care of a birth parent within a year.
- However, over the next five years, *two thirds of those will have a further period in care* which, for the majority, will become a long-term arrangement.
- This means that, at the end of the five-year follow-up period less than a third of children initially received into foster care are still living with their birth parent but only half of those who will eventually move into alternative care on a long-term basis appear to have been identified during their first care episode.

The evidence therefore suggests that care planning (i.e. multi-agency decision-making about the right placement for the child) is of crucial importance. Thinking about our example, there may have been very sound reasons for sending the 'subsequent returners' home after their first experience of foster care. But it also raises the possibility that our methods for identifying risk and averting subsequent harm may be no more reliable than tossing a coin.

There are few published studies which have systematically studied children as they experience repeated changes of home and care-giver. An exception is Tarren-Sweeney's longitudinal research which has demonstrated a relationship between number of placements and later mental health, although this is difficult to disentangle from age at entry to care: those children who had multiple placements also tend to be those who entered care for the first time at an older age and tend to have poorer mental health (Tarren-Sweeney, 2008). We suggest that there are at least two ways in which repeated placements may be problematic. First there is good reason, both on theoretical grounds and from related studies (Lewis et al., 2007), to expect that children exposed to such experiences will be at greatly increased risk of attachment insecurity. And second, given that these children have, by definition, experienced repeated exposure to maltreatment in the birth family, the risks of other trauma-related mental health difficulties is also increased. Clinical work with looked after and accommodated children in Glasgow has, therefore, developed a focus on informing care planning with the aim of improving child mental health.

In many parts of the UK, child and adolescent mental health services (CAMHS) have begun to adapt and develop the way that they provide services for children and young people who live in the care of their local authority. In Glasgow, two particular strands of clinical work were introduced: one ('LACES') offered a dedicated, easy-to-access CAMHS service for children and young people with emerging and established mental health difficulties; the other (Routine Psychological Assessment [RPA]), designed for younger children when they first come into care, was set up using early intervention principles (Dimigen et al., 1999) with the aim of promoting resilience and reducing the risk of mental health problems emerging.

Given the absence of a well-evidenced model of care specific to either population, the team adopted a systemic approach to service development. Here the models of care would adapt through successive iterations, informed by the slowly growing evidence base and in light of feedback received from the people who used the service as clients and as colleagues.

Both clinics soon found that the well-recognised models of assessment and formulation which they were using had to be adapted to take cognisance of a *care-planning domain*. Members began to report that care-planning issues sometimes appeared directly related to the clinical issues under consideration. Curious about this possible relationship, members began to ask social work colleagues about this. For example, what did s/he think about a foster carer's account of coincidence between episodes of disturbed behaviour and a child's contact (supervised visits) with a birthparent whose violence the child had described to the carer?

Over the course of many such discussions, team members recognised that, while in some cases care plans appeared robust, well evidenced and in the child's best interests, there was a significant minority where this was not the case. In these, various aspects of care-planning could contribute to placement instability, to further trauma or both. This happened readily when the case was being 'twin-tracked'. This refers to a situation where the authority believes that a child is likely to need alternative care but takes the view that does not have sufficient evidence to make the legal case. This 'twin-tracking' approach is a de-facto arrangement in contrast to 'Concurrent Planning' which is enshrined in legal statute and requires system change for full implementation (Frame, Duerre Berrick, & Foulkes Coakley, 2006). In the 'twin-tracking' approach, the care-plan proceeds as if preparing for the child to go home, for example with increasing contact with biological parents, while the authority monitors the process for further evidence which would create a legal basis for permanency, potentially exposing the child to further harm. Over time, the team in Glasgow has consolidated these observations into its formulation model and therefore reports now routinely address themselves to the specific question of the likely impact of the care-plan on the child's mental health.

It is important to acknowledge at this stage that in most countries, including the UK, decisions about the permanent placement of maltreated children are made, not by local authorities but by the judiciary, with assessments by social workers and/or clinicians providing advice to inform these decisions. The outcome of that advice depends on how it is perceived and regarded by those who are party to the decision, and occasionally the judiciary decides to send a child home even when the local authority is recommending permanency. If mental health considerations are to inform such decisions, practitioners have to recognise that acceptance can depend upon the disposition of both the local authority and the local judiciary. Although the judicial systems in England and Scotland with regard to permanency are very different, the mean age of adoption in both countries is around 4 years (http://www.gro-scotland.gov.uk/press/news2004/03adopt-press.html; http://www.baaf.org.uk/info/stats/england.shtml), so we are not achieving early decisions in either country.

Why is early intervention with maltreated children so important?

The first few weeks and months of life are time of most rapid brain growth and development (Huttenlocher & Dabholkar, 1997). The human brain is immature at birth, compared to other primates, and this may be because the development of many of its most important functions (e.g. complex social interaction) are dependent on interaction with adults (Blaffer-Hrdy, 1999; Trevarthen & Aitken, 2001). Lack of interaction with adults, such as happens in the context of neglect or the fearful withdrawal that result from an atmosphere of violence, deprives the young infant of the environment necessary for normal development. Maltreatment can have permanent and profound effects on the developing brain, particularly the areas involved in stress responses, memory functioning, attention, language, planning and social interaction (Teicher et al, 2003).

The effects of maltreatment on the complex stress response system are particularly important. The cerebral cortex is rich in receptors for stress hormones and is therefore particularly susceptible to the negative effects of maltreatment. One of the roles of the cortex is to have an inhibitory effect on the stress response system (the hypothalamic-pituitary axis) (Teicher et al., 2003) so maltreatment can set in train a vicious cycle of effects where the child becomes even more vulnerable to the stressful situation they are being raised in (Essex, Klein, Cho, & Kalin, 2002; Fairchild et al, 2008). Research has shown that maltreated toddlers are at risk of having abnormal diurnal patterns of production of the stress hormone cortisol (Dozier et al, 2006a). This is particularly important because abnormalities of diurnal cortisol production have been shown to be associated with conduct problems and antisocial personality disorder (Fairchild et al, 2008).

The story is not a wholly negative one, however. Because the structure of the human brain is not fixed, remarkable change can take place particularly in the early months and years of life (Hosking & Walsh, 2005). Mary Dozier has shown that an intervention (Attachment and Biobehavioural Catch-up) which trains carers to be extra-nurturing with maltreated toddlers can return their abnormal stress responses to normal patterns (Dozier et al, 2006b; Dozier, Peloso, Lewis, Laurenceau, & Levine, 2008). Even children exposed to extreme social and emotional deprivation, such as those raised in the orphanages of Ceausescu's Romania, can achieve remarkable recovery in growth, cognition, mental health and social behaviour when placed in family care (Nelson, Zeanah, & Fox, 2007; Nelson et al, 2007; Zeanah, Smyke, Koga, & Carlson, 2005).

Maltreated children can rapidly develop secure attachments when placed in the care of a sensitive and secure foster carer, regardless of the severity of their behaviour problems (Dozier, Stovall, Albus, & Bates, 2001; Stovall-McClough & Dozier, 2004). The security of attachment in foster care is also related to the degree of commitment of the caregiver to the child: in other words, if a foster carer considers the placement to be temporary, the child is less likely to develop a secure attachment than if the caregiver sees herself as having a lifelong caregiving role (Lindhiem & Dozier, 2007).

Unsurprisingly, placement instability such as we see in many local authorities in the UK has a detrimental effect on mental health (Delfabbro & Barber, 2003; Newton, Litrownik, & Landsverk, 2000), so the sooner good decisions can be made about where a young maltreated child will spend the rest of his or her life the better. In 1997, the US Federal Government introduced the Adoption and Safe Families Act, which aimed to prevent maltreated children being returned to unsafe homes and to 'expedite permanency' in safe, loving adoptive homes where necessary. If a child has been in care for 15 of the last 22 months, a permanency decision should be made. There is some evidence that the ASFA is increasing the rates of adoption (Gendell, 2001) but there are also concerns that the time pressure on permanency planning may have negative consequences in some instances (Phillips & Bloom, 2009). The decision about whether to return a child to a family in which s/he has previously been maltreated or to place him or her permanently in an adoptive family is a momentous one. We must find ways to make timely informed decisions and to test whether or not we make the right ones.

The New Orleans intervention

In New Orleans, a group of clinicians and scientists – the Tulane University Infant Team – have developed and evaluated an intervention (Zeanah et al, 2001) which helps to ensure appropriate and timely decisions about permanent placement of maltreated children. In Jefferson Parish in Louisiana, every child under the age of 5 years who has been validated as having experienced maltreatment and placed in foster care is referred to the team for evaluation and treatment. Following referral, the Infant Team embarks on a detailed attachment-based assessment. Beginning with each foster carer, the process goes on to include each member of the child's family – including non-biological partners – who is directly involved in care-giving. This leads to an intervention with the birth family aimed at maximising the chances of the child returning to their care:

> The intervention team attempts to define explicit treatment goals and to design specific interventions to help parents achieve those goals within a time frame that is reasonable for the children ... . The *sine qua non* of treatment goals is helping parents accept responsibility for their children's maltreatment. From this overarching goal, all other specific goals and interventions derive.
>
> (Zeanah et al, pp. 215–6)

The intervention is offered in all cases on the premise that the outcome in relation to parental responsibility cannot be predicted reliably from the information available prior to the intervention. The course of the intervention also contributes significantly to the body of evidence necessary to make the case for termination of parental rights to the judiciary, where the course of the intervention indicates that this is in the child's interest. The intervention involves evidence-based programmes tailored to the needs of the family such as Circle of Security (Cooper, Hoffman, Powell, & Marvin, 2005) or Child-Parent Psychotherapy (Lieberman, Ippen, & Van Horn, 2006). These focus on the attachment and wider relationship between the birth parent(s) and the child and aim to improve parent–child interaction.

A number of features differentiate the New Orleans Model from the typical approach to maltreated children and their families in the UK: first, intensive intervention is offered in every case: the purpose of assessment is to allow the intervention to be tailored to the individual case; second, foster carers are usually jointly registered as adopters so that children remaining in care can stay with the same family; and third, the decision about permanency has to be made within around 15 months or less. This model extends the concept of Concurrent Planning in that it offers 'concurrent intervention'. Zeanah, the director of the team, and his colleagues have evaluated the New Orleans Model by comparing routine childcare data in the four years before and after the programme began. It has resulted in an increased number of children freed for adoption, but where children were returned to the birth family, there has been a reduction in subsequent incidents of maltreatment of that child and of subsequent incidents involving siblings (Zeanah et al., 2001).

The team in New Orleans are convinced of the need for thorough assessment through structured interviews, self-report measures and observations which assist in identifying the child's developmental and emotional needs in the context of maltreatment. In Charley Zeanah's words, they elicit '*a sense of what's happening interactionally and then what's happening subjectively*'. The work identifies parallel areas where intervention should occur, between child and foster carer and child and biological parents. The planned intervention also addresses the problems which the parents are experiencing. So assistance with, for example, substance abuse, mental health issues and domestic violence are all built into the intervention which is co-ordinated by the Infant Team.

The Infant Team identify a number of factors which are related to a good outcome, one of which, accepting responsibility for the maltreatment of children, is of central importance, with change represented by learning from interventions to become 'a safe and effective parent'. While there is an assumption that the child will be returned to the parents, this is not always possible and the aim of the model is to have 'the best outcome possible for [the] particular child'.

Could such a model be implemented in the UK? This would depend, to a large extent, on the will of clinicians, social workers, policy makers and the legal profession to make fairly radical changes in approaches and attitudes towards permanency planning for maltreated children. Implementation is likely to be complex and we have therefore decided to adopt an evidence-driven approach to instituting and managing the development of a 'New Orleans Model' service in Glasgow: A 'Complex Interventions' approach. This approach to developing interventions that consist of several inter-related parts – in other words complex interventions – was first developed by the UK Medical Research Council (Campbell et al., 2000). The model suggests that an innovative intervention be developed in overlapping phases which take account of the context in which the intervention is being implemented and the existence of multiple components which need to be understood (Campbell et al., 2000). The overall aim of this approach is to optimise the intervention itself and the methods of evaluating it before deciding whether a definitive study, ideally a randomized controlled trial, is necessary (Campbell et al., 2007).

We have begun such an approach to evaluating the implementation of the New Orleans model in Glasgow. In this chapter, we describe part of the 'mapping and modelling phase' (Campbell et al., 2000) in which we have used qualitative techniques to investigate the way the intervention works in the New Orleans context and the potential barriers and drivers supporting or preventing successful implementation in Glasgow. We set out to ask:

- What are the key components of the New Orleans model as practiced in Louisiana?
- How similar/different are the clinical, social and legal contexts in New Orleans and Glasgow?
- What might be the added value of implementing the New Orleans model in Glasgow?
- How might it be implemented in Glasgow?

Translating the model for Glasgow

In April 2009, three members of a Glasgow 'implementation team' (a child and adolescent psychiatrist and two social workers) made a five-day visit to New Orleans. They took with them a list of questions for the New Orleans team that had been prepared in advance in consultation with the Glasgow steering group. Seven key interviews and meetings with New Orleans staff and one meeting of the Glasgow steering group, upon their return, were audio-recorded. All audio-recordings were transcribed verbatim and an independent rater, with clinical experience in child and family mental health, conducted a qualitative analysis of their content.

Analysis

In consideration of the research questions, the independent rater was required to explore how individuals discuss translation of the model in addition to what was emphasised as important for the clinicians in their work (e.g. values, aims and approaches). In line with phenomenological approaches, each transcript was examined in detail noting reflections and preliminary themes. Emerging themes were then clustered for each transcript to capture a sense of the whole narrative process and categories were developed. By going through the transcripts a number of times, phrases, repeating patterns, differences between transcripts and so on, were identified and new themes were acknowledged (Smith & Osborn, 2003). Themes were then clustered under super-ordinate themes in a thematic table with each transcript reviewed again by cutting and pasting excerpts. The analysis was therefore cyclical, requiring movement between the independent rater and the text, noting agreement and tensions in each transcript. Discussions with two Glasgow team members regarding the development of the coding framework aimed to enhance credibility.

Translation themes

From the meetings in New Orleans and Glasgow two main themes emerged. The first theme reflected discussions between the New Orleans and Glasgow teams about *'wanting what is best'* for infants in foster care, with discussions focusing on the purpose of the work and the challenges associated with working in such complex systems. These discussions reflected much shared knowledge and professional experience of working with maltreated children and their families and also highlighted the processes necessary to distil and articulate clearly the needs of the children so that the right decisions can be made regarding their future. The second theme *'preparing for change'* illustrates the finer details regarding the application of the model in Glasgow. This theme derived mainly from discussions between the Glasgow team and the agencies who work alongside the Infant team in Louisiana to support the delivery of the service.

Wanting what is best for the child

This theme embraced a range of topics relating to professionals' experiences of working with looked after and accommodated children and the intention for all of wanting what is best for the child.

Working within constraints

Respondents shared frustrations in achieving the best outcomes for the child and their sense of powerlessness in relation to the systems in which the child lives. For both the New Orleans team and the Glasgow team there was a view that the needs and best interests of the children carry relatively little weight when decisions are made. By contrast, both teams spoke of factors such as the quality of relationships between social workers and parents critically influencing decisions regarding permanency or termination of placements. As one New Orleans team member remarked sardonically:

> "I think that children don't vote – children have very little power."

Seeing the whole picture

This theme highlights the emphasis placed by both teams on developing a clear view of all of the key elements in a complex system and communicating on the strength of that view. As one New Orleans worker stated:

> I think we meet families and see the dynamics, we see psychopathology, we see family history, we see all of it, and we figure things out faster than the rest of the system.

This complexity is illustrated by the way relationships between the agencies and families influence and shape the assessment task and yet the workers have to find ways of representing the work done dispassionately. Professionals discussed working with ambiguity and how they each go about managing this, referring to the importance of continually constructing and re-constructing a picture of a family and the progress they make. One of the New Orleans team members gave a particularly telling illustration of the dilemmas which arise when she said:

> You're constantly working with your client towards getting them to be the parent they need to be and at the same time monitoring all of the reasons why they're not there yet ... then you need to write the report to court.

The implications of seeing the whole picture meant that workers felt a strong sense of responsibility in being the 'holder' of a child's history, a perspective which resonated strongly with the concern, already noted, of the difficulty of 'making children's voices heard'. Members of both teams noted that thorough assessment, informed by available evidence and based on the whole picture, played a key role in achieving the best outcome for the child. The New Orleans team experience has been that such assessments enable the right decisions to be made.

Making the right decisions

Workers felt empowered by evidencing practice and the recommendations that can be made on that basis. For the Glasgow team members, the prospect of structured assessment and planned intervention provided optimism.

GLASGOW TEAM MEMBER: 'I think that's where its power lies ... (being able to say) that we have arrived at this outcome, having given a very reasonable and sustained shot at making it work. One of the tricky things about an assessment-only type service is that you're saying, "based on our assessment, we're saying this shouldn't happen or it should happen"'.

For the Glasgow team, hearing New Orleans team members' stories consolidated the concept of not just intervention, but also prevention of future maltreatment of children. As another Glasgow team member noted:

> [in Glasgow] you don't give enough opportunity for people to have (a) therapeutic experience, and therefore quite often children do go into drift because parents come back.

The content of this theme also linked to a sense of the Glasgow team preparing themselves for change, imagining what the model would look like for their families.

Preparing for change

GLASGOW TEAM MEMBER: 'We're here because of our experience being unsatisfactory ... this is about learning to do something different.'

Much of this theme derives from discussions held in the Glasgow steering group with clinicians, social workers, researchers and managers. What resonates throughout this theme is the *'spirit of New Orleans'* (Glasgow team member) with individuals drawing on stories and experiences from New Orleans, with a firm emphasis on *'making the right decision'* for the child.

Preparing others for change

As one New Orleans team member noted, in order to influence the decisions that are made about an innovative service, you have to be able to sell it:

> you can get a brand name that carries some clout.

In engaging others in this process of change, Glasgow team members felt it was important for there to be a sense of transparency about what the model would look like for children in Glasgow. As such, extensive discussion was devoted to the practicalities of applying the model and consideration of the skills and support mechanisms needed to put it in place locally.

Skills and support

From discussions in New Orleans, it was noted that having therapeutic experience was an essential requirement for working in the Infant team, but professionals would draw upon 'training specific' rather than 'discipline' specific skills. Different members of the New Orleans team have expertise in particular areas e.g., Child-Parent Psychotherapy (Lieberman et al, 2006), Circle of Security (Cooper et al, 2005) and so on and it appears that decisions regarding interventions are made as a team, matching skills and experience to each case and clarifying an ethos of non-hierarchy.

GLASGOW TEAM MEMBER: 'the fundamental thing [in New Orleans] is that [they] have far better-evidenced assessments with an obvious clear programme of work with the parents ... and we do not have that at the moment.'

Discussions in Glasgow in turn mapped staff required for the new Glasgow team, based on what was deemed essential in New Orleans and what is practical or feasible in Glasgow.

Practicalities of employing the model

There are a number of possible requirements for the model to work in Glasgow. One of the major practical challenges is having a legal system which supports the model. In New Orleans there is a direct relationship with the court system. As mentioned earlier, this is not the case in Scotland. But this was not seen as an insurmountable barrier in the following discussion within the Glasgow team:

GLASGOW TEAM MEMBER 1: 'Is the legal situation in Scotland so different from that in Louisiana that comparability and fidelity would be impossible? I don't think so. But I just think you have to have it working. Do you have to have the working model of the whole thing before you can actually work that out?'

GLASGOW TEAM MEMBER 2: 'No. I don't think we can. We'll not know. I think what we have to do is see if we can get as good a deal with the legal system as we can.'

Discussion

With reference to our research questions, the Glasgow team came back from New Orleans with a sense of understanding key components of the model, including concrete information about structured assessments, measures and interventions and more abstract information about the philosophy of the team. The team were keen to communicate the essence of the 'spirit of New Orleans' to Glasgow colleagues and there was much discussion on their return about how best to 'sell' the model to key stakeholders.

Some aspects of the clinical, social and legal contexts were surprisingly similar in the two locations: both the New Orleans and Glasgow teams felt frustrated by barriers to delivering an equitable service to children and were preoccupied by attempting to ensure that the needs of the child are prioritised, clarified and valued. These similarities highlighted the Glasgow team's perception that there was a gap in our ability to provide an assessment and treatment approach which is both holistic and which provides clear and timely recommendations that can be taken on by colleagues in the legal system.

An important question arises as to whether a Glasgow version of the programme in a different legal context would be a different intervention. There are divergent views about whether or not evidence-based programmes should be adhered to with absolute fidelity or whether local modification is necessary or even desirable (Hawe, Shiell, & Reilly, 2004). There is a body of expert opinion that local adaptation of a model may be necessary but 'investigators need to be clear about how much change or adaptation they would consider permissible' (Craig et al, 2008, p. 14).

What might be the added value of implementing the New Orleans model in Glasgow? There was an excitement about the possibility that the New Orleans model offered a framework and skills that could be transferred to the Glasgow context and could improve practice. There was a sense that the model could facilitate Glasgow workers' abilities to provide the kind of holistic yet clear portrait of the child and of the birth family's ability to change, allowing the right decisions to be made. On return to Glasgow, discussion soon turned to details of local implementation, with attention ranging from staffing complement and skills required through to organisational supports and permissions required. An early objective in this phase would be taking the first steps in getting the model accepted by local stakeholders. This may well be a legitimate focus at this early point in the journey: the process of introducing a change in clinical practice is a challenging one and issues such as how to win over opinion leaders who disagree with evidence, or influence clinicians who are too busy to appraise the evidence require careful consideration (Grol & Grimshaw, 2003).

An exploratory randomised controlled trial of the 'Glasgow Infant and Family Team' is currently underway. Our qualitative mapping and modelling exercise has helped us shape our ideas about how to make the service a reality, and has also helped us develop a shared clarity about where we are in the long process of testing its effectiveness in practice.

Note

1 This chapter was previously published as: Minnis, H., Bryce, G., Phin, L., & Wilson, P. (2010). The 'Spirit of New Orleans': translating a model of intervention with maltreated children and their families for the Glasgow context. *Clinical Child Psychology and Psychiatry*, 15(4), 497–509.

References

Blaffer-Hrdy, S. (1999). *Mother Nature*. New York: Chatto and Windus.

Campbell, M., Fitzpatrick, R., Haines, A., Kinmonth, A.L., Sandercock, P., Spiegelhalter, D., (2000). 'Framework for design and evaluation of complex interventions to improve health'. *British Medical Journal*, 321, 694–696.

Campbell, N.C., Murray, E., Darbyshire, J., Emery, J., Farmer, A., Griffiths, F., [(2007). 'Designing and evaluating complex interventions to improve health care'. *British Medical Journal*, 334, 455–459.

Cooper, G., Hoffman, K., Powell, B., & Marvin, R. (2005). 'The circle of security intervention: Differential diagnosis and differential treatment'. In L.J. Berlin, Y. Ziv, L. Amaya-Jackson, & M.T. Greenberg (Eds.), *Enhancing early attachments: Theory, research, intervention, and policy* (pp. 127–151). New York and London: The Guilford Press.

Craig, P., Dieppe, P., McIntyre, S., Michie, S., Nazareth, I., & Petticrew, M. (2008). 'Developing and evaluating complex interventions: The new Medical Research Council Guidance'. *British Medical Journal*, 337, a1655.

Delfabbro, P.H., & Barber, J.G. (2003). 'Before it's too late: Enhancing the early detection and prevention of long-term placement disruption'. *Children Australia*, 28, 14–18.

Dimigen, G., Del Priore, C., Butler, S., Evans, S., Ferguson, L., & Swan, M. (1999). 'The need for a mental health service for children at commencement of being looked after and accommodated by the local authority: questionnaire survey'. *British Medical Journal*, 319, 675.

Dozier, M., Manni, M., Gordon, M.K., Peloso, E., Gunnar, M.R., Stovall-McClough, K.C., (2006a). 'Foster children's diurnal production of cortisol: an exploratory study'. *Child Maltreatment*, 11, 189–197.

Dozier, M., Peloso, E., Lewis, E., Laurenceau, J.-P., & Levine, S. (2008). 'Effects of an attachment-based intervention on the cortisol production of infants and toddlers in foster care'. *Development and Psychopathology*, 20, 845–859.

Dozier, M., Peloso, E., Lindhiem, O., Gordon, M.K., Manni, M., Sepulveda, S., (2006b). 'Developing evidence-based interventions for foster children: An example of a randomized clinical trial with infants and toddlers'. *Journal of Social Issues*, 62, 767–785.

Dozier, M., Stovall, K.C., Albus, K.E., & Bates, B. (2001). 'Attachment for infants in foster care: The role of caregivers state of mind'. *Child Development*, 72, 1467–1477.

Essex, M.J., Klein, M.H., Cho, E., & Kalin, N.H. (2002). 'Maternal stress beginning in infancy may sensitize children to later stress exposure: effects on cortisol and behavior'. *Society of Biological Psychiatry*, 52, 776–784.

Fairchild, G., van Goozen, S., Stollery, SJ., Brown, J., Gardiner, J., Herbert, J., (2008). 'Cortisol diurnal rhythm and stress reactivity in male adolescents with early-onset or adolescence-onset conduct disorder'. *Biological Psychiatry*, 64, 599–606.

Frame, L., Duerre Berrick, J., & Foulkes Coakley, J.F. (2006). 'Essential elements of implementing a system of concurrent planning'. *Child and Family Social Work*, 11, 357–367.
Gendell, S.G. (2001). 'In search of permanency: A reflection on the first 3 years of the Adoption and Safe Families Act Implementation'. *Family Court Review*, 39, 25–42.
Grol, R., & Grimshaw, J. (2003). 'From best evidence to best practice: Effective implementation of change in patients' care'. *The Lancet*, 362, 1225–1230.
Hawe, P., Shiell, A., & Reilly, T. (2004). 'Complex interventions: How "out of control" can a randomised controlled trial be?'. *British Medical Journal*, 328, 1561–1563.
Healthcare Commission (2009). *Review of the involvement and action taken by health bodies in relation to the case of Baby P*. London: Healthcare Commission.
Hodges, J., & Tizard, B. (1989a). 'IQ and behavioural adjustment of ex-institutional adolescents'. *Journal of Child Psychology and Psychiatry*, 30, 53–75.
——(1989b). 'Social and family relationships of ex-institutional adolescents'. *Journal of Child Psychology and Psychiatry*, 30, 77–97.
Hosking, G., & Walsh, I. (2005). *The wave report: Violence and what to do about it*. England: Wave Trust.
Huttenlocher, P.R., & Dabholkar, A.S. (1997). 'Regional differences in synaptogenesis in human cerebral cortex'. *Journal of Comparative Neurology*, 387, 167–178.
Lieberman, A.F., Ippen, C.G., & Van Horn, P. (2006). 'Child-parent psychotherapy: 6-month follow-up of a randomized controlled trial'. *Journal of the American Academy of Child & Adolescent Psychiatry*, 45, 913–918.
Lindhiem, O., & Dozier, M. (2007). 'Caregiver commitment to foster children: The role of child behavior'. *Child Abuse & Neglect*, 31, 361–374.
McCann, J.B., James, A., Wilson, S., & Dunn, G. (1996). 'Prevalence of psychiatric disorders in young people in the care system'. *British Medical Journal*, 313, 1529–1530.
Meltzer, H., Gatward, R., Corbin, T., Goodman, R., & Ford, T. (2003). *The mental health of young people looked after by local authorities in England* (Rep. No. The report of a survey carried out in 2002 by Social Survey Division of the Office of National Statistics on behalf of the Department of Health). London: The Stationery Office.
Minnis, H., Reekie, J., Young, D., O'Connor, T., Ronald, A., Gray, A., et al. (2007). 'Genetic, environmental and gender influences on attachment disorder behaviours'. *British Journal of Psychiatry*, 190, 495.
Nelson, C.A.I., Zeanah, C.H., & Fox, N.A. (2007). 'The effects of early deprivation on brain-behavioral development: The Bucharest Early Intervention Project'. In D. Romer & E.F. Walker (Eds.), *Adolescent psychopathology and the developing brain: Integrating brain and prevention science* (pp. 197–215). Oxford: Oxford University Press.
Nelson, C.S., Zeanah, C.H., Fox, N.A., Marshall, P.J., Smyke, A.T., & Guthrie, D. (2007). 'Cognitive recovery in socially deprived young children: The Bucharest Early Intervention Project'. *Science*, 318, 1937–1940.
Newton, R.R., Litrownik, A.J., & Landsverk, J.A. (2000). 'Children and youth in foster care: Disentangling the relationship between problem behaviours and number of placements'. *Child Abuse & Neglect*, 24, 1363–1374.
O'Connor, T.G., & Zeanah, C.H. (2003). 'Attachment disorders: Assessment strategies and treatment approaches'. *Attachment and Human Development*, 5, 223–244.
Phillips, S., & Bloom, B. (2009). 'Permanency planning in the context of parental incarceration: legal issues and recommendations'. In C. Seymour & C. Finney

Hairston (Eds.) *Children with parents in prison* (pp. 75–92). Piscataway, NJ: Child Welfare League of America.

Smith, J.A., & Osborn, M. (2008). 'Interpretive phenomenological analysis'. In J.A. Smith (Ed.) *Qualitative psychology: a practical guide to research methods* (2nd edition ed., pp. 53–80). London: Sage.

Stovall-McClough, K.C., & Dozier, M. (2004). 'Forming attachments in foster care: Infant attachment behaviors during the first 2 months of placement'. *Development and Psychopathology, 16*, 253–271.

Tarren-Sweeney, M. (2008). 'Retrospective and concurrent predictors of the mental health of children in care'. *Children and Youth Services Review, 30*, 1–25.

Teicher, M.H., Andersen, S.L., Polcari, A., Anderson, C.M., Navalta, C.P., & Kim, D.M. (2003). 'The neurobiological consequences of early stress and childhood maltreatment'. *Neuroscience and Biobehavioral Reviews, 27*, 33–44.

The Highland Council (2009). *Dundee Child Protection Committee: Significant Case Review – Brandon Lee Muir*. Dundee: The Highland Council.

Trevarthen, C., & Aitken, K.J. (2001). 'Infant intersubjectivity: Research, theory, and clinical applications'. *Journal of Child Psychology & Psychiatry & Allied Disciplines, 42*, 3–48.

Wilson, P., Bryce, G., Puckering, C., & Minnis, H. (2008). *Parenting Services for Children in Glasgow Discussion Document*. Unpublished report for NHS GG+C Director of Public Health.

Zeanah, C., Smyke, A., Koga, S., & Carlson, E. (2005). 'Bucharest early intervention project core group: Attachment in institutional and community children in Romania'. *Child Development, 76*, 1015–1028.

Zeanah, C.H., Larrieu, J.A., Heller, S.S., Valliere, J., Hinshaw-Fuselier, S., Aoki, Y., (2001). 'Evaluation of a preventive intervention for maltreated infants and toddlers in foster care'. *Journal of the American Academy of Child and Adolescent Psychiatry, 40*, 214–221.

6 Social-emotional screening and intervention for 0–4-year-old children entering care

Carol Hardy and Elizabeth Murphy[1]

Summary

The subject of this chapter is our attempt to look more closely at 0–4-year-old children in the care system, and to describe a pilot service that aimed: to identify their social-emotional needs quickly; to promote their development and attachment to their caregivers; and to contribute towards better care planning. We will discuss what led us to identify this need and describe the context in which this work developed. We will describe the social and emotional screening and intervention service that we implemented for 0–4-year-old children in care to an inner-London Local Authority. For each of the stages of this we will discuss process issues with the implementation of the screening and mention the limitation of the work.

Introduction

Rationale for the screening and intervention

The threshold for taking children into care is very high and many 'looked after' children have only been removed from their families after years of abuse and neglect. When infants enter the care system therefore, their circumstances are often particularly extreme and they are at their most vulnerable; completely dependent on a safe adult/caregiver. These early years are a critical time for emotional and neurological development (Schore,1994, 2001) which is highly dependent on the care of an adult who can recognise, think about and respond to the infant's and young child's needs. Children and young people who become looked after by local authorities are among the most vulnerable and disadvantaged in society (Sempik, Ward, & Darker, 2008). They are at increased risk of poor outcomes for child and adult mental health, educational attainment, employment and criminality (Ford, Vostanis, Meltzer & Goodman, 2007; Davidson, 2008).

We know that Children in Care (CiC) are still not receiving services in a timely fashion (Ward, Holmes, Soper & Olsen, 2008). In modern times, CiC have often experienced traumatic events in their lives, so it is unsurprising that they are more likely to develop mental health problems than those in stable family environments, with all the attendant disadvantages for their development and well-being. A survey in England found that 45% of CiC aged 5–17 years had a mental health disorder. This is five times more likely than children in private households (Meltzer, Corbin, Gatward, Goodman, & Ford, 2003). Even though these children are a high risk group for mental health disorder they often go unrecognised and untreated (McMillen et al, 2005; Mount et al, 2004).

It is mostly older CiC who receive CAMHS interventions and even then many of their needs are overlooked (Whyte & Campbell, 2008). Data for children entering care in England in 2005-2006 showed that 35% of this group were 0–4 years. However, little is written on children under 4 in care and there is a call for more research with this group (Sempik et al, 2008; Milburn, Lynch, & Jackson, 2008). In England there are longstanding concerns about poor permanency planning for CiC across the age range (Rowe & Lambert, 1973; Department for Children, Schools and Families, 2002). Children who are removed from their families following severe and enduring abuse and neglect, then face the possibility of additional adversity in care, including drift in care planning, placement changes, poor relationships and educational attainment, which further increases their risk of developing mental health difficulties (Tarren-Sweeney, 2008).

Generally in England, babies and young children who enter Local Authority care are initially placed with short-term, temporary carers while the decision about their long-term care plan is worked out in court. It is usual that there are delays in the court process because of the need to obtain expert assessments and the care proceedings being contested. Short-term carers thus often become medium- to long-term carers, and the child's needs can be overlooked as the decisions about the permanency plan for the child remain unclear.

The commitment to the child from a caring adult is very different depending on whether you see yourself as a long-term or short-term carer. One of the strongest indicators that a child will become securely attached is foster carers' positive attachment and commitment to the child (Dozier, Stovall, Albus, & Bates, 2001; Dozier & Lindhiem, 2006). Reviews of social care data (Ward et al, 2008) shows the timeframe for decision-making about long-term care for infant and children is far longer than the six months suggested. Social Care services are often subjected to repeated and often last minute demands by the courts to carry out additional assessments and as the short-term carer becomes a medium-term carer for a growing child who is beginning to express their frustration, confusion and anger. This 'drift' puts pressure on the placement. There are usually high levels of contact between the birth parents and the infant during the court proceedings (as frequent as four times a week). Research and reviews of this contact show that the contact is often not in the best interest of the infant (Kendrick, 2009; Schofield & Simmonds, 2011). The infant experiences uncontained and inexplicable disruption and this can further inhibit the development of relationships between foster carers and infants. All parties may end up feeling aggrieved – none more so than the child who in this process is truly a hapless victim. Foster carers may feel justified in asking for the child to be moved to another foster home and sadly in many cases the cycle of repeated placement breakdown begins. In our clinical experience very few children stay with the carer they were first placed with or go on to be adopted by their foster carers.

It is a mandatory requirement in the UK for all CiC to have regular health checks by a general practitioner (G.P. i.e. a family physician) or paediatrician. However, it is not a requirement that all CiC have a routine *mental health* check. We know from clinical experience that we need detailed profiling of the child's development, along with their interactions and relationship with the carer to identify need and inform intervention. Even if there is agreement about assessing the emotional/mental health needs of the infant, mental health assessment of under 4s is a contentious area. How can one best capture a child's mental health disorder(s), and given the child's age and developmental needs also consider their difficulties and strengths in the context of past and current relationships between the child and their caregivers?

While reviewing the numbers of children in care with the local authority we realised that there were a high number of under 5s who remained in care and were not being referred to our service. Given we are a bespoke CAMHS team serving one local authority's CiC population, we wanted to investigate why there was a low referral rate for 0–4s and to what degree there was an unidentified and unmet need about the social emotional and mental health needs of looked after children aged 0–4 years. We added an intervention component as evidence from previous screening studies showed that recommendations from screening led to children receiving CAMHS input in only a small proportion of cases (Burns *et al*, 2004).

Early patterns of attachment interactions are established in the first few days/weeks (Stovall & Dozier, 2000) of a child being placed with a new carer so it is crucial that this is looked at in detail early in the child's life in care. With infants and children the earlier the intervention the greater its chance of success because of the child's receptivity and capacity for change.

National context

In the late 1990s and early 2000s, the British government recognised the plight of children in care and the failure of the system to offer mental health intervention in a timely way. Under 'Quality Protects' money many child and adolescent mental health services were established specifically to address the needs of looked after children. These were influential developments that helped ensure more effective multi-agency management and delivery of services and appropriate assessment, intervention and support for these children. However, this did not achieve all that is necessary.

In England, policy and practice about permanency planning for CiC has been debated for decades with concern about the quality of care plans for CiC, and drift in decision-making where time and considered planning is of the essence (Goldstein, Freud & Solnit, 1973; Performance and Innovation Unit, 2000; Department for Children and Families, 2002).

Alongside this, the National Institute for Clinical Excellence (NICE) and the Social Care Institute for Excellence (SCIE) recently published a public health guide for looked after children (NICE, & SCIE, 2010). It specifically identified the needs of under 5s and stressed the need to 'ensure all babies and young children are assessed by a specialist child mental health worker to ensure the child does not exhibit signs of emotional distress (for example children or babies who may exhibit passive, withdrawn or over compliant behaviour)'. It also asked that services 'offer early and preventive interventions for babies and young children to avoid placement breakdown and reduce the impact on a child's potential to develop meaningful relationships in the longer term'. In his national review of early intervention, Graham Allen argues that service delivery should move from late reactionary to early intervention for the under 5s (Allen, 2011). There is an acknowledgement about the plight of the 0–4s in policy along with the difficulty of transforming service delivery and clinical practice.

Local context

The present screening and intervention project took place at Carelink, the Southwark Child and Adolescent Mental Health team (CAMHS). This multidisciplinary team, which is co-located with the Local Authority Social Care team, offers assessment and treatment to children and young people in the care of Southwark Social Care. The team has strong links with Social Care and Child Health and so at both a strategic and operational level have support to ensure buy-in across the service to help overcome barriers and gain cooperation in the implementation of this pilot. This inner London local authority is densely populated and many of the foster carers live outside the Borough. Over 50% of children seen in the Carelink team live outside the Borough. This has implications for service delivery.

Purpose of the study

In this study we set up a pilot service to screen the emotional/social development and mental health needs of all children 0–4 years entering the care of an inner London Local Authority in 2010 to 2011 with funding secured from the Guy's and St. Thomas' Charity. As part of the screening we also provided a brief intervention for the child's carer and advice to the professional network where a need was identified. We carried out evaluation to see if this screening process was effective, and to use the data collected on the level and

Social-emotional screening and intervention   103

type of needs found to inform us about the development of more comprehensive and effective services.

In a separate paper (in preparation) we have described the method, data analysis and results in detail.

The screening/intervention service in practice

In this section we will describe the main stages of the service, starting each with a brief description of the activity involved, and following this with a commentary on how it worked and was developed in practice.

'Getting started' – Introducing a new system

Southwark social services provided a weekly list of children who had become looked after and were waiting to have an initial health assessment (IHA) with a community paediatrician. Once an IHA had been scheduled, an information sheet was sent out to the birth parent, foster carer, child's social worker and 'supervising social worker' (a social worker from the Fostering team supporting the foster carer) letting all those concerned know that we would join the IHA to start the screening process unless the birth parents exercised their right to opt out of the study.

Commentary

To get this initial stage of the project underway we needed the close cooperation and trust of colleagues in both Social Care and Child Health, so that we had access to these confidential data. Discussions had begun well before the project start date with senior clinicians and managers to ensure the smooth running between different departments including Administration, I.T, Health and Social Care teams across the borough.

The project staff also visited Referral & Assessment, Fostering and CiC teams to describe the procedure and respond to questions and anxieties that professionals raised. Overall the project was greeted with interest by staff, whilst also conveying a strong sense of how pressurised they felt for time. An anxiety was expressed that foster carers would be criticised. These meetings helped us to be mindful of the perceptions of foster carers and professionals alike and shaped our approach and communication with them at all stages of the process. Specific examples will be given in the following sections regarding the different tasks and demands on our participants.

'Meet and Greet' – first steps in engaging our participants

The birth parents (if present), the child and foster carers were met for the first point of direct face to face contact at the Initial Health Assessment

(IHA) in the Child Health clinic. The IHA's were generally organised for 4 weeks following the child's entry into care.

The rationale for using the IHA for the initial contact was two-fold: firstly that it was part of an existing routine procedure that we could join, to meet the carer and child early on and complete the standardised questionnaire; and secondly there would be the opportunity to gather information on the child's developmental assessment through discussion with the Paediatrician.

The project information sheets were available in case the carer/parent had not received the copy sent by post or if they wished to have another copy on the day to ask questions about specific points.

Commentary

The majority of carers and birth parents had not read the information sheets or newsletter before the IHA, so we had to work quickly to engage them in conversation and describe the project in a sentence or two, letting them know they could take time to consider, with the choice to opt out. By adopting this approach we found that some parents who initially refused at the IHA, later agreed to their child taking part. Only four parents refused outright for their child to be screened, resulting in 94% uptake of participants into the project.

Although not planned with this in mind, we thought that the first point of contact being in Child Health did help the carers/parents alike to engage with us, as a 'doctor's clinic' was a familiar setting for the adults. Importantly too, it is likely that the participating adults sensed the cooperation between the professionals. We experienced a growing ease with which we and the paediatricians found a way to share the space of the medical, whilst the doctors got on with their primary tasks.

Although counterintuitive considering the young age of our sample, we found that to a large extent the baby and toddlers were the easiest participants to engage with, in that many displayed a complete lack of discrimination when meeting us or the paediatricians in the reception area.

> A common example of this would be as follows. As we sit down to talk with an unfamiliar foster carer, Child A, aged 18 months, walks round to my knee and leans against me, actively trying to engage with smiles. The doctor calls the group into clinic and she marches off without a backward glance to her carer, leading the group of adults down the corridor.

Integrating child development and health assessment into the social-emotional screening – 'not a case of either/or'

In the majority of cases the research worker and/or the CAMHS clinician would observe the child whilst the Paediatrician conducted the health and developmental assessment, being sensitive to occasions when the birth

Social-emotional screening and intervention 105

parent wanted time alone with the doctor. Informal observations were made and recorded.

Commentary

Many more benefits than expected emerged over time by joining the IHA. We had the opportunity to see how the child functioned in an unfamiliar setting, the uncertainty and anxiety for the child compounded at times by the sudden appearance of their parent(s) and a degree of tension felt by foster carers and birth parents alike. We noted the extent to which the carer and/or birth parent(s) could facilitate the child to settle and engage in the activities and examinations, a marker of how much they could put the needs of the child first and withstand the pressures of the environment.

The observations of the child with the paediatricians gave valuable insight into the potential of the child's functioning and developmental levels, sometimes demonstrating a greater capacity to engage with and master play tasks than seen later on the home visits, or the reverse being true where we noted the child to perform differently in the home environment. Many times we saw babies and children being drawn out by the skill of the paediatrician.

> Baby B, aged 9 weeks was described by his birth mother, with whom he was in a Mother-Baby Assessment Unit, as being unresponsive and sleepy for the majority of the day and night. The paediatrician evoked an interest and willingness on the baby's part to engage in lively face to face interaction, leading to B trying to engage his mother in this way, albeit unsuccessfully as the mother was unresponsive. This information, when fed back to the Social worker, led to her approaching the baby differently and a heightened awareness of the baby and indeed mother's capacities.

We had the opportunity to observe a wide range of behaviours and responses from the babies and children that contributed useful material towards our developing formulation and ongoing conversations with carers e.g. the eagerness on a child's part to learn, and equally those children who were more preoccupied/anxious, hyper-vigilant and easily distracted by any noise, fearful of failure, or sensitive to their perception of this from the adults.

At times during the IHA there would be the opportunity for straightforward conversations between ourselves and the paediatrician on the child's presentation which was helpful in thinking with the carers about the emerging difficulties, and how we might plan to address these as a first step. When this was not possible we would often consider our combined observations and thoughts afterwards in making plans, e.g. the timing, number and type of services to refer a young child to in the context of them having disrupted daily routines with contact, numerous appointments to attend or considerable time away from their foster carer if nursery places had been introduced.

'Usefulness of Parent/Carer report questionnaires' – integrating standardised questionnaires with clinical assessment

The appropriate standardised questionnaire for the age of the child was completed in or immediately after the IHA. If there was insufficient time in the IHA, this was postponed to the home visit. Both the Ages and Stages: Social and Emotional (ASQ:SE) (Squires, Bricker & Twombly, 2003) and the Greenspan Social and Emotional Growth Chart (SEGC) (Greenspan, 2004) questionnaires were administered in most cases as a semi-structured interview unless a parent chose to complete it independently. We will focus here on examples from the ASQ:SE as this is a more comprehensive questionnaire.

Commentary

Incorporating the questionnaire into a wider conversation about the carer's or parent's view of their child gave the opportunity for the foster carer or parent to expand on specific questions, giving examples of the child's responses in different situations. Importantly too, it provided information about behaviours where the carer felt that the child rarely showed a behaviour or not sufficiently often as they would expect for a child's age/developmental level. In these instances the behaviour would obtain a score of '0', indicating 'no concern' from the questionnaire alone. By administering the questionnaire like a clinical interview we gained useful insights into both the child's strengths and the type of adaptive behaviours or coping strategies they had developed.

> Child C, a 2 year old girl, was presenting with feeding difficulties (gorging food, no awareness of being full and tearful whenever she saw adults eating) along with temper tantrums outside of the foster home. However she scored below the clinical cut off on the ASQ:SE due to a high level of self-reliant behaviour. This child had delayed expressive language but the carer could reflect on how little Child C would communicate on a non-verbal and emotional level in a wider discussion.

Two critical factors became apparent that were influencing the low scores that many of the children gained from administering the ASQ-SE. The first of these was the positive wish on the carer's part to present the baby/child in 'a good light'. Often in these instances there would be hesitation on the carer's part to some questions and more exploration would reveal a real underlying concern they held about the child's lack of response e.g. not seeking comfort when hurt. In other scenarios we initiated a discussion where there was a sense that the carer had come to accept the child's unresponsiveness or passivity as the norm. The second factor was the actual prevalence of undemanding, passive and withdrawn behaviours in our sample. The latter contributed to the finding that 55% of babies and children over 3 months scored below the standardised cut off point on the ASQ:SE, as few difficulties were raised from the questionnaire alone. However, in this same group of children over 3 months, 66% of babies/children went on to be recommended an intervention, as we found that specific concerns became known through discussion with the carer and/or later observations of the child–carer interaction.

Some common themes that emerged through more in-depth questioning included carers distinguishing between children who could comment on adults' emotional states yet had no words to describe their own feelings, children who would accept cuddles, with more of a sense of tolerance than enjoyment or comfort, and who equally would never initiate or indicate a need for any physical contact.

> Child D, a four year old boy, was initially described by the carer as loving hugs and affection, thereby scoring '0' points on this question in the ASQ:SE. During the intervention the carer acknowledged her difficulty in providing nurture for this child who refused comfort by standing with his arms rigidly by his side.

The scores and descriptive examples provided evidence of behavioural change that had already taken place, giving insight into how the child had responded to the foster carer, and equally what may be behavioural indicators that an individual child is under stress.

> Child E, aged 15 months, who was controlling, unable to focus and had frequent screaming outbursts including head banging when first looked after; these behaviours reducing over the first few weeks with carer. However this information was noted in the screening report so that consideration could be given to their possible re-emergence at future significant transitions.

Observations of child–carer relationship in the home

A home visit was arranged after the IHA to complete the Parent Caregiver Involvement Scale (PCIS) (Farran, Kasari, Comfort, & Jay, 1986) which was specifically chosen as the standardised observational measure, because it includes important dimensions of a carer–child relationship that we were interested in exploring further, whilst being brief and non-intrusive to administer. The observation is not videoed, thereby making the visit as comfortable as possible for the carers. Occasionally we met resistance to the home visits, when times were cancelled or repeatedly difficult to arrange, and more liaison was needed with social work colleagues in Fostering or CiC teams as social workers and carers questioned our reason for seeing babies and children at such a young age.

The visits were completed by both the research worker and Clinical Specialist in the majority of cases as this gave us the chance to regularly test our inter-rater reliability for the measure, as well as having a second pair of eyes, especially useful when visiting a busy and active sibling pair. Informal observations were made and recorded under the same categories as at the IHA. If the foster carer left the room, or there were any other notable stressors during the visit, the child's response was recorded.

Commentary

In general we had a positive response to our visits to the carers' homes, with both foster parents and kinship carers alike. Having already met most of the carers at the IHA, we had begun to develop a shared interest and language about the individual child. As there was a wide variance in the range of carer's backgrounds, including their experience, ethnicity and age, it was important to be open to and respectful towards their individual circumstances, while also finding ways to sensitively introduce some of our ways of thinking about and understanding the children. We were acutely aware of the recent distressing situations that the babies and children had experienced before entering care, and the emotional burden of this that the carers were absorbing, albeit unconsciously at times.

In their own homes, away from the tensions of sharing a space with birth parents in the IHA, we wanted to see what was possible in the newly developing relationship between carer and child. Overall this led to rich and helpful insights into the experience and functioning of the baby/child, as well as illustrating how quickly patterns of interaction become established (Stovall & Dozier, 2000). Sometimes this was a joy to witness as the carers had clearly embraced the child into their home and emotional world. At other times we could see carers working very hard to care for and become close to children who remained remote and subtly unresponsive to these efforts. We saw situations in which the child and carer had already developed a more didactic relationship, in which the carer resorted to largely instructing the child to carry out certain behaviours or activities and little emotional warmth or reciprocal interaction was evident.

> Child F was 15 months old at the time of the home visit, and had scored well below the standardised cut off on the ASQ:SE. As we sat with her and her carer, who were playing together on the floor, we initially observed how much she looked around, seemingly interested in the toys. Her carer made many efforts to chat and engage her. As the observation progressed we noted that she was never in any physical contact with her carer and, although increasingly tired, did not signal a

Social-emotional screening and intervention 109

wish or attempt to be close to her. When the period in which the PCIS observation took place had ended, we explored this with the carer. She explained that the child had no need of her, making her feel quite rejected. Through discussion we articulated that a pattern had become established by which the carer felt defeated in her attempts to nurture this child. This carer was open to thinking more about the impact of this on their relationship, and the reasons why this may have come about. It helped her to resume her natural caregiving responses. We had seen ourselves how quietly but determinedly this baby pushed her away to remain alone and self-soothe. Live and shared experiences like this are powerful and can help with engaging carers.

Screening summary report

The information from the IHA, screening questionnaires, home visit observations, developmental and health information from the paediatricians, and background information was considered and written into a screening summary by the CAMHS Clinical Specialist. This included a formulation and recommendations for the child's social and emotional development. This was distributed to the child's social worker, foster carer, paediatrician and independent reviewing officer (IRO). The summary was sent in time for the next Looked after Child Review meeting (LAC Review) so that the information could be incorporated in the consideration and discussion of the child's needs. (LAC reviews in the project area take place at 1 and 4 months following a child entering care and are key decision-making forums focusing on the specific needs and of the child.)

Commentary

In designing the template for the screening summary, thought was given to factors that would ensure busy professionals and carers would read and digest its contents. The report needed to be brief and succinct (two sides only), have accessible language, i.e. avoiding clinical jargon, to predominantly describe the child's presentation rather than include carer observations, and to include clear indicators for what kind of intervention was needed.

Although it was inevitably easier to write the summary reports when the carer was clearly articulating problem child behaviours, it was necessary to include some observations and these were carefully worded. We frequently needed to highlight the fact that the difficulties centred on there being an absence of expected responses from the child to the carer. Some initial hypotheses were made about contributing factors to this if there were strong indicators of impact from antenatal drugs/alcohol, general or specific developmental delays or high levels of contact described as distressing to the child. Although necessarily tentative, these thoughts helped pave the way for further conversations about the baby or child's experience before entering care, which at times were painful for the carers. With kinship carers we were mindful of the particular emotional conflicts that family members may have in thinking about what the child had experienced in the care of their own close relative.

The summary would always include some positive statements about either the child's strengths and/or progress along with an acknowledgement of particular ways in which the carer was intervening or being thoughtful about the child. These comments were specific so that they would resonate with the carer and make them feel we had taken note of their efforts and experience of caring for the child.

The report was usually sent to the professionals in the network, but given in person to the carers along with the opportunity to discuss the content and its implications for further contact with the project where this was indicated. This gave us the chance to engage the carer in thinking about their contribution being of the greatest importance in effecting change for the baby/child. It could be more challenging to elicit a carer's involvement if they felt that the child was 'doing fine' or was 'no trouble' and at times we had some work to do in influencing colleagues that an intervention was needed.

Where the summary report pointed to the child progressing positively and having no specific concerns, this account was also welcomed by the IRO and network. There was a standard reminder at the end of each report that the screening was not a full CAMHS assessment and that anyone could request further assessment if they thought this necessary. Occasionally a social worker, having found the initial summary helpful, would ask for a review sooner than our 6-month follow-up.

> Baby G, aged 4 months, and her birth mother had left the residential assessment unit and returned home after a few weeks. The review screening contributed to the interagency monitoring and recommendations made for the mother, who had an older child looked after at the time.

Decision-making following screening

When an intervention or advice to the foster carer or network was indicated from the screening findings we had follow up conversations or meetings with the child's social worker to agree the planned intervention. These always included the fostering social worker and foster carer for the child.

Commentary

Our plan to convene a meeting to discuss the screening and to plan the intervention was the one aspect of the project where a lower level of activity occurred than we had anticipated as it was difficult to quickly secure times which all the relevant people could make. We then made a decision whether to sacrifice the meeting to keep the momentum and engagement with the carer and avoid delay for the intervention. A pragmatic approach was adopted and we liaised informally with the child's social worker at times. Meetings often took place as the intervention came to a conclusion and we needed to consider what was needed next.

It could be argued that the screening process and feedback formed an assessment and intervention. In some instances the sharing of screening information resulted in immediate decision-making regarding the care planning for the child.

> Child C's care plan (a 2 year old girl described earlier) was changed when the summary report was distributed and the decision made by social care to delay her return home until CAMHS work had begun. The project team facilitated this referral and mother and child were seen together for sessions before and after Child C had been rehabilitated home.

Type and level of interventions offered

As our primary goal in this exploratory project was to see if we could recruit families, carers and professional networks to engage with the screening, we had not set out firm parameters for the interventions – in part as we were yet to find out the scale and diversity of the children's needs and difficulties in their social-emotional development and capacity to relate to their caregivers. We had asked for funding which would make provision for two face-to-face follow-up meetings with the carer and child but not been prescriptive about the precise format for the intervention. The thinking around having this flexibility was the experience from our existing referrals that the baby/child presentations could vary widely and we wished to respond with an individualised package of care according to the needs identified. We therefore took the approach of implementing what was most helpful and viable in each instance. In most cases this resulted in direct work with the carer alongside liaison and advice to the network. We noted how much and what type of intervention was taken up in each case from the list below:

- Liaison with professionals
- Network meeting including foster carer to discuss screening assessment
- Advice on social-emotional needs of child to foster carer (individualised advice sheets)
- Direct guidance and support to foster carer/network professionals
- Direct carer–child work

Commentary

Most of the options listed were being used in our clinical response to referred cases before the project, with the exception of the written advice sheets which we developed during the project as an adjunct to direct support and advice to carers. Clinical experience of working with high risk under fives, including CiC, meant that treatment approaches focusing on the carer–infant/child attachment and developmental guidance had been developing over some years. At their core are early infant mental health and child development principles, attachment theory and the belief that the carer–child relationship is the main agent for change. From the many approaches developed in parent/carer–infant work (Fraiberg, 1994; Lieberman & Van Horn, 2008) we have a body of knowledge to draw on to help when addressing the disturbed and disturbing nature of these babies' manner of relating to others. Stern's (1995) notion of therapy approaches 'utilising different ports of entry into a single dynamically interdependent system' is helpful as it recognises the complex variables, behavioural and representational, that are at play in the system of the carer–child relationship, but also provides a framework to consider the starting point for the intervention. This was particularly relevant in this project where we had a very short timeframe to engage carers, children and professionals to reflect and act differently with the child's emotional states and needs. We also were dealing with a wide variety of circumstances of different legal status, babies and children being cared for by birth mothers, close relatives, local authority or agency foster carers, and a wide geographical area. This both challenged and influenced our decision-making on how to maximise the screening information into a helpful intervention in the individual situation for each child. As is often true in clinical work, 'no one size fits all'.

Specifically to foster children, the core concepts in Mary Dozier's Attachment and Biobehavioural Catch-Up treatment approach (Dozier, Bick, & Bernard, 2011) have both informed and have common ground with our clinical work with foster carers, especially the carer's need to override a tendency to respond to the child's signals that they have no need of nurture or care as if this was real, and to address the carer's uncomfortable feelings about providing nurture to distressed babies and young children.

> Baby H was 11 months when first seen at the IHA. He had spent his early months with his parents at home. Their relationship had been violent, with both partners as perpetrators of attacks on the other. Birth mother was looked after herself as a child due to her own family's problems with violence and alcohol abuse. Baby H on entering care was underweight and dirty with dry skin. He showed no response to being separated from his parents at the point of removal, nor when the regular contacts with parents ended. He seemed indifferent to who he was with and settled immediately into the foster home and routine there.
>
> His carer completed the ASQ:SE and he scored few points, indicating little or no concern for his development. He was described as smiley with good eye contact and yet the carer described that he had a 'remote' feeling about him, that he seemed uninterested in interacting with

others. He would not let the carer know if he was hurt and did not check where she was if they were around strangers.

As we thought about how self-contained he was, he banged his head hard against the door and walked away immediately, picking up a toy. When I commented on what had happened to him he looked around with a fixed smile but began to grimace as if registering the pain and upset. This led to a peculiarly distorted facial expression, as if one emotional state was merging with another. He regained control quickly and the fixed smile gained precedence again. His avoidant style was equally reflected in the relationship between him and his carer. The carer could speak about the existence and strangeness of this phenomenon but had become distanced herself from the feelings and capacity to register the emotional state of the baby.

The work began by having a joint meeting with the child's social worker and foster carer. We discussed the screening report and approaches that actively addressed his avoidance and the lack of reciprocal communication between them. The carer was responsive to the plan to meet together with Baby H to try out new ways of relating with him using the live interaction between them. In this instance the carer's representations of the child were gently explored alongside support to persist in offering care to this 'reluctant' baby and reflection on the emergence of new cycles of interaction. Anxiety that was raised in the process within both carer and child could be thought about, along with the pace of change. This carer, like some others, questioned their perception that they were 'forcing' the child to relate differently, particularly as physical contact was involved. Whilst recognising the need to be sensitive to the feelings that are evoked in these very young children, the work needs also to address ambivalent feelings on the carer's part without them feeling criticised or pushed too quickly into difficult emotional territory.

When the core pattern of relating had begun to change, this gave a foundation from which to think about other more specific behaviours that Baby H was presenting with. These included being slow to respond to verbal communications (so much so that it raised concern that he was deaf) and a controlling and almost compulsive approach to tidy and hide his toys.

Although there wasn't scope within this project to use attachment classification measures we were conscious of how many young children had experienced very frightening and unpredictable events and the prevalence of children presenting with extremely controlling behaviours suggestive of a disorganised attachment response. As with Baby H, these behaviours were accommodated by the carer who put his more obsessional behaviour down to an inevitable inherited response from his birth father. The intervention revealed how much H could relinquish these behaviours when he had developed an emotional dependence with his carer.

In a few cases where interventions were recommended but not taken up by the network, we were subsequently asked for consultation and intervention for the children and carers in the weeks following the end of the project.

Feedback from the network – views from carers and professionals across the agencies

After each screening a feedback questionnaire was sent to the child's social worker, IRO, paediatrician and foster carer asking for their feedback on the screening summary and with the foster carers, their experience of the screening process. In the cases where an intervention was recommended and implemented we sent the questionnaire out following the end of the intervention period.

Commentary

Of the 63 children who took part in the study, we obtained feedback from at least one person involved in their care in 90% of cases. In response to questions about the screening summary, 98% of participants reported that the screening summaries were 'clear and helpful'. IROs regularly commented on how helpful the reports were for the child's LAC review and would contact us close to the reviews to check that a report was on its way.

We asked the social workers to say how the screening had influenced their decision-making around care planning, direct work with the child, and/or with the carer. Positive responses to each of these were at 45%, some social workers stating that it helped their thinking when speaking with carers/birth parents and interacting with the children themselves. The mixed response to how much it influenced care plans was as a result of social workers' view that the outcomes were being strongly driven by court assessments, or by the likelihood that the child would eventually be placed for adoption or remain with a close relative.

The response to the interventions was consistently positive, with carers' ratings on a 5-point scale (with '5' being the highest rating) resulting in a mean score of 4.6, and the social workers' feedback giving a mean score of 4.3.

To some extent the feedback also reflected the professionals' experience that the parents' view takes precedence over the needs of the child, especially in this group where so many are preverbal or too young to express themselves clearly. One foster carer said 'I am the voice for this baby'. We shared this sentiment, and worked hard alongside others to make the children's feelings and experience heard.

Reviews

After six months, children who remain in care receive a review health assessment (RHA) by the paediatrician. Although not an original goal of the project we decided that where possible a repeat of the initial screening was completed at the RHA including observation of the child during the assessment and completion of the ASQ:SE with the foster carer. If this was not possible at the RHA the research worker arranged a home visit, or a convenient time for a phone conversation, to complete the ASQ:SE with the foster carer.

Commentary

Children who were screened in the first eight months of the project were reviewed, and we achieved this in 74% of cases. Where it was not possible to arrange a review, the children had either returned home or had become subject to a Special Guardianship Order.

Although we did not have time to repeat all the measures we had completed in the initial screening, we gathered enough information to be able to report on the child's progress or where new or changing needs had become known. The Adoption Panel was particularly interested and keen to receive screening summaries. In cases where children were followed up with a referral made to our CAMHS CiC team, we have gone on to share both the screening and subsequent work with the child with the adoptive parents themselves. This still continues for those children screened later in the project who are at the point of moving to adopters now.

Conclusion

In the year prior to the pilot of this new screening/intervention service, social-emotional concerns were identified in 10% of 0–4-year-olds entering care, and referrals made as a result of this did not include ones to the CiC CAMHS team. In contrast, during the year when the screening took place, 67% of the screened population were highlighted with specific concerns and recommended an intervention with the CAMHS Clinical Specialist. We had the opportunity to see the majority of the 0–4 CiC in the pilot year due to the high uptake of participants (94% of the eligible population). If anything, the level of need identified is likely to be an under representation as it is difficult to accurately screen babies under three months of age, applicable to over a quarter of our sample.

The procedure devised for this screening project was well received and proved acceptable to a wide range of carers and professionals. This was achieved partly through the screening process striking a balance between a standardised method along with some flexibility and clinical assessment to engage carers and children. An essential component at all stages was our strong interagency relationships that could be tested at times in the context of competing demands. Considerable time and effort was needed to highlight the children's needs as well as consider the impact from court, contact and care planning procedures.

With the increasing interest shown in the individual screening reports and interventions came also a heightened awareness and thought for the babies/ young children's emotional experience and development. We heard how this impacted on professionals' own practice as well as on concrete care plans for the child and over time we received requests for not only reviewing children who were in the project but to also extend this service to children who were not new to care. Whilst a one-year project is limited in following and reviewing children, we think this work has gone some way to exploring the unrecognised difficulties in these young children and raised the perspective of their experience.

For the future we can see developments of this model to more closely involve birth parents, to develop stronger evidence about the most effective interventions, and to review these children's progress and needs over a longer time period. We have described both an opportunity and a practical process by which we can help give 'a voice' to vulnerable babies and young children entering care along with the work with and support for carers. This work extends across the many transitions these babies and children make moving to adopters, long-term carers or return to birth parents when reflections on the past and hopes for the future continue to resonate.

Note

1 We would like to express our appreciation for the support provided by the Guys and St. Thomas' Charity that made the work described here possible. We are grateful too for the support and collaboration of paediatric colleagues in Child Health, especially Dr Beatrice Cooper, research colleagues Elizabeth Hackett and Susan Conroy, our many social care colleagues and to the foster carers and children.

References

Allen, G. (2011). *Early Intervention: The Next Steps*. The Stationery Office, London.

Burns, B., Phillips, S., Wagner, H., Barth, R., Kolko, D., Campbell, Y., & Landsverk, J. (2004). 'Mental health need and access to services by youths involved with child welfare: A national survey'. *Journal of the American Academy of Child and Adolescent Psychiatry* 43, 960–970.

Davidson, J. (2008). *Children and Young People in Mind: The Final Report of the National CAMHS Review*. London: DCSF.

Department for Children, Schools and Families. *Adoption Guidance: Adoption and Children Act 2002*. London: DCSF.

Dozier, M., Stovall, K.C., Albus, K.E., & Bates, B. (2001). 'Attachment for infants in foster care; The role of caregiver state of mind'. *Child Development*, 72, 1467–1477.

Dozier, M., Bick, J., & Bernard, K. (2011). 'Attachment-based treatment for young, vulnerable children'. In J. Osofsky & A. Lieberman (Eds.), *Clinical Work with Traumatized Young Children*. New York: Guilford Press.

Dozier, M., & Lindhiem, O. (2006). 'This is my child: Differences among foster parents in commitment to their young children'. *Child Maltreatment*, 11, 338–345.

Farran, D., Kasari, C., Comfort, M., & Jay, S. (1986) *Parent/Caregiver Involvement Scale*. Vanderbilt University.

Ford, T., Vostanis, P., Meltzer, H., & Goodman, R. (2007) 'Psychiatric disorder among British children looked after by local authorities: comparison with children living in private households'. *British Journal of Psychiatry*, 190, 319–325.

Fraiberg, S., Ed. (1994). *Assessment and Therapy of Disturbances in Infancy*. London: Jason Aronson Inc.

Goldstein, J., Freud, A., & Solnit, J. (1973). *Beyond the Best Interests of the Child*. New York: Free Press.

Greenspan, S. (2004) *The Greenspan Social Emotional Growth Chart: A Screening Questionnaire for Infants and Young Children*. Oxford: Pearson Assessment.

Kendrick, J. (2009). 'Concurrent planning: A retrospective study of the continuities and discontinuities of care and their impact on the development of infants and young children placed for adoption by the Coram Concurrent Planning Project'. *Adoption and Fostering*, 33(4), 5–18.

Lieberman, A.F., & Van Horn, P. (2008). *Psychotherapy with Infants and Young Children*. New York: Guilford Press.

McMillen, J.C., Zima, B.T., Scott, L.D., Auslander, W.F., Munson, M.R., & Ollie, M.T. (2005). 'Prevalence of psychiatric disorder among older youths in the foster care system'. *Journal of the American Academy of Child and Adolescent Psychiatry*, 44(1), 88–95.

Meltzer, H., Corbin, T., Gatward, R., Goodman, R., & Ford, T. (2003). *The Mental Health of Young People Looked after by Local Authorities in England*. London: The Stationery Office.

Milburn, N., Lynch, M., & Jackson, J. (2008). 'Early Identification of mental health needs for children in care: A therapeutic Assessment programme for Statutory Clients of Child protection'. *Clinical Child Psychology and Psychiatry*, 13(1), 31–47.

Mount, J., Lister, A., & Bennun, I. (2004). 'Identifying the mental health needs of looked after young people'. *Clinical Child Psychology and Psychiatry*, 93(3), 363–382.

NICE, & SCIE. (2010). *Promoting the Quality of Life of Looked-after Children and Young People: Public Health Guidance PH28*. London: NICE / SCIE.

Performance and Innovation Unit. (2000). *Prime Minister's Review of Adoption*. London: Cabinet Office.

Rowe, J., & Lambert, L. (1973) *Children who Wait*. London: Association of British Fostering Agencies.

Schofield, G., & Simmonds, J. (2011). 'Contact for Infants subject to care proceedings'. *Family Law*, 617–622.

Schore, A. (1994). *Affect Regulation and the Origin of the Self: The Neurobiology of Emotional Development*. New Jersey: Lawrence Erlbaum.

——(2001). 'Effects of secure attachment on right brain development, affect regulation and infant mental health'. *Infant Mental Health Journal*, 22, 7–66.

Sempik, J., Ward, H., & Darker, I. (2008). 'Emotional and behavioural difficulties of children and young people at entry into care'. *Clinical Child Psychology and Psychiatry*, 13(2), 221–233.

Squires, J., Bricker, D., & Twombly, E. (2003) *The ASQ:SE User's Guide*. Baltimore: Paul Brookes.

Stern, D. (1995). *The Motherhood Constellation*. New York: Basic Books.

Stovall, K., & Dozier, M. (2000). 'The development of attachment in new relationships: Single subject analyses for 10 foster infants'. *Development and Psychopathology*, 12, 133–156.

Tarren-Sweeney, M. (2008). 'Retrospective and concurrent predictors of the mental health of children in care'. *Children and Youth Services Review*, *30*(1), 1–25.

Ward, H., Holmes, L., Soper, J., & Olsen, R. (2008). *Costs and Consequences of Placing Children in Care*. London: Jessica Kingsley.

Whyte, S., & Campbell, A. (2008). 'The strengths and difficulties questionnaire: A useful screening tool to identify mental health needs in looked after children and inform care plans at looked after children reviews?'. *Child Care in Practice*, *12*(2), 193–206.

7 Using an attachment narrative approach with families where the children are looked after or adopted

Rudi Dallos and Annie Dallos

Attachment theory has contributed much to our understanding of how children develop emotional connections and bonds to their parents. For children who have been separated from their biological parents and find themselves with substitute carers, either through the looked after children system or more permanently through adoption, the process is considerably more complex. For the majority of these children, the attachment process involves managing simultaneously the loss or availability and connections with their birth parents as well as the forming of new bonds with their new carers. Others may have to manage multiple disruptions and changes of care givers before moving into a more permanent placement.

From his original observations of children in looked after contexts, Bowlby (1979) identified how separation from a child's attachment figure could lead to an inability to trust others in order to form secure and lasting relationships. He suggested that all children developed a set of expectations from their prior experiences about whether adults could be trusted and to what extent the world generally was a safe as opposed to unsafe place. Specifically this included expectations about the extent to which the child felt that they could rely on others or essentially had no one but themself. He called this the child's 'internal working model', and this was seen to operate both at a conscious, but perhaps most influentially, at an unconscious level, to shape how we act. The core feature of the working model is that it constitutes a set of strategies for how the child tries to ensure safety from danger. At its most fundamental the child requires the parents to keep them physically safe, remove the distress of hunger and discomfort and also to provide emotionally intimacy and support.

Studies of children and young people in care have shown that they generally hold insecure, and in many cases, complex traumatic attachment representations (Crittenden, 2008; Tarren-Sweeney, 2010). Foster placements and adoptive placements are often fraught with difficulties for children and carers alike with frequent breakdown occurring (Steele et al, 2003; Tarren-Sweeney, 2010) and children suffering further disrupted attachments. Freyd et al (2011) identified that foster placement breakdown was most likely for young people showing dissociative symptoms: 78% of looked after children will have been abused and neglected and a large proportion display some symptoms of PTSD, and many programmes of treatment for 'attachment disordered' children focus on managing the influence that trauma has had on their lives.

In contrast children who have secure working models hold a view that parents are physically and emotionally available when they need them. They also regard themselves as worthy and deserving of affection, and believe their parents understand and appreciate their needs. This generates a mutual sense of being 'held in mind', and of caring about each other's feelings and needs, along with a sense of connection and ability to positively influence each other's actions. This has also been called inter-subjectivity – a sense of mutual connection and ability on the child's part to influence their parent (Treverathen & Aiken, 2001; Hughes, 2007). Arguably, even children who were secure before an adoption process might struggle and would benefit from support.

Children who have experienced trauma through disrupted attachments may instead have developed a sense that others do not consider their feelings, that they cannot influence others and subsequently they may abandon attempts to consider the feelings of others. An unfortunate consequence may be that they come to be experienced negatively by their carers, as being withdrawn, overly self-reliant, self-centred, lacking the desire for intimacy, superficial, risk-taking and relationally shallow. Attachment theory suggests that in fact internal models and the strategies which they guide, are 'functional' and are acquired in order for the child to survive in the particular family environment they are in (for example, to avoid being hurt further, either emotionally or physically). Whilst the defences associated with the strategies served a survival function early in life, they are no longer necessary for their physical or emotional well-being and can become counter-productive in the new potentially safer context with their carers. Unfortunately, in some cases the child's representations may also become self-fulfilling. For example, it is hard for children to relax when they feel a constant need to control their environment; and this habit of hyper-vigilance can prevent a child or young person from recognising that he or she is now in safe hands. Their continuing anxiety, suspicion and withdrawal may reduce the opportunities for them to feel secure and experience feeling cared for and thus confirm their sense of isolation, anxiety and anger.

Foster carers and prospective adopters will typically have been educated about the emotional needs of the looked after child through specially designed programmes which aim to inform them about the impact of disrupted attachments and abuse on children. In our experience invariably these may not sufficiently prepare the carers for the emotional challenges they may have to manage themselves. In some cases it can lead to a misguided view that they are in some way responsible for 'fixing the child' when a more realistic goal is to provide an environment in which the child can gradually develop a degree of trust and security. The therapeutic challenge is

Using an attachment narrative approach 121

to enhance parents' positive emotion, instil hope, increase parents' motivation, and create a more effective model through which to view their parenting role and understanding of their child. Aiming for more modest goals which recognise the difficulties and challenges involved, can help to avoid the sense of failure and distress that some carers come to experience.

In this chapter we draw from our work with families in a community-based Family Therapy Service in the South West of England and with families worked within our independent practice, Family Focus. We begin by considering the passage below from the first meeting in a course of family therapy with two adoptive parents, Brenda and Mark and their two adopted sons, Carl (17) and David (11):

RD (TO MARK): Do you feel that sometimes he thinks you don't care or don't love him?
MARK: I don't know. I know that I am extremely peed off with him. Because it's eight years we have had him, seven years of absolute crap (tears in his voice. Brenda touches his knee for comfort). Police, police, running away, phoning social services, stealing, smoking, drinking, drugs dealing. (to Carl) ... I've tried to talk to you, I'm peed off, unhappy, I love you, I don't think you want to be part of the family (tears in his voice)
MUM: That's how actions speak but I don't know why ...
MARK: I don't think you're sorry, you've got no remorse, when you're doing it, about the family, I see your brother crying when you do things like that. You say you love him, I think you don't. I've seen your mum in bits ... you're a good kid but you really need to ... Take charge of yourself, otherwise you're gonna be in drugs, jail and probably dead. And it ain't anything I can do. I'm angry (nodding head)
RD: Thanks for being honest
MARK: I am honest. I just don't know what to do (tearful)
RD: Is it like this at home, that you have this conversation?
MARK: Yes, I am angry with him
CARL: We don't really talk (tearful)
MARK: We don't talk, we don't do nothing
CARL: I push people away (tearful)
BRENDA: I don't know how much goes back to the early years ... was told he needs a strong male role model. Wish he could get that into his head

Mark and Brenda will have been aware that young people entering adoption may be suffering from a wide range of problems and disadvantages, including conduct disorders and defiance, disorders of mood such as anxiety and depression, anti-social behaviour including criminal behaviours, educational under-achievement, and difficulties in forming relationships. Yet in the family conversation above we hear Carl's adoptive father Mark list many of these behaviours as if he was in some way both surprised and devastated that the love and stability they have offered him and his brother through adoption does not seem to be enough. A sense of failure and lack of confidence in 'not being up to the job' is an experience shared by most parents at different times in their parenting, not only foster carers and adopters. However, the meaning of this will be different for adopters who may come to the task already with a sense of failure, if for example they have been unable to have their own children. Furthermore, their motivations may be shaped by corrective scripts (Byng-Hall, 1995; Dallos, 2006) featuring attempts to do parenting differently to how their own parents were with them. Children are often unaware of the corrective scripts guiding their parents' strategies and are instead likely to experience their parents' sense of frustration and dismay as similar to their prior experiences of anger, abuse and rejection from their previous attachment figures.

We have found that the carers' resilience may be more dependent on their own attachment histories than their professional knowledge about the needs of attachment disordered children. Attachment research indicates that half of the general population (UK, N. America and Europe) have experienced an insecure attachment in their own childhoods and that the proportion of insecure attachments of people in the caring professions exceeds that of the average population (Van Izjeson et al, 1992; Cassidy and Shaver, 2010). Given this distribution, it is highly likely that many foster carers and adopters will also have developed insecure attachment strategies as a way of managing their own insecure childhood experiences. Individuals are most likely to employ these coping strategies when under threat, therefore it is not surprising that they are not always clearly evident during an assessment process but may become more apparent (as in the family above) when children in placement activate them through some of the severe emotional challenges that their behaviour poses to their carers.

It may be seen as a financial drain on agencies and experienced as intrusive for carers to have formal attachment assessment at the recruitment stage. Nevertheless, we have found that when placements are at risk of breakdown, most carers find it helpful to look at their own attachment strategies, for example by engaging in a full or partial Adult Attachment Interview (AAI). This can help to offer areas for reflection with them to guide and support therapeutic intervention. Such explorations reveal that parents who have experienced a secure attachment themselves do not generally feel as emotionally threatened by the complex behaviours, rejections, anger and withdrawal that many adopted children display. Even in this case though, there are differences, and carers may differ in terms of whether they display an 'earned' as opposed to 'naïve' secure pattern. In the former the parents have experienced adversity, conflict, anger and deception but have learnt to resolve these experiences. They therefore appear to have a more robust set of coping strategies. Parents who have consistently experienced care and nurturance may be a little more surprised and unbalanced by a child who displays such complex and challenging behaviours, such as deception, lying, stealing, inconsistency and so on. In a similar vein, parents who hold insecure strategies, for example a parent who has experienced rejection themselves as a child and consequently developed an attachment strategy that avoids intimacy and comfort, may find their previous ways of coping with this triggered by the rejection from the child for whom they are caring. In many cases this is compounded by the carer's corrective scripts whereby they are wishing to do things differently to their own parents, for example to be more emotionally warm and responsive. Subsequent experience of rejection of these attempts may lead them to doubly feel they are failing and also that the child does not appreciate their intention to do things better. This cocktail of a sense of failure, exasperation, feeling unappreciated and so on, can in turn contribute to the child's insecurity, further provoking insecure responses from the carers.

Tracking such patterns of entangled emotional responses by drawing them out as relational patterns or circularities (Dallos and Draper, 2010) has become a core feature of our model. Returning to the extract above, we can see that Mark describes the concerns they have about the risks that Carl is taking, for example with drugs, staying out and his choice of friends, culminating in their fear that if Carl continues his ways of acting he may end up dead. Brenda starts to express awareness of how Carl's early experiences, before his adoption by them at the age of eight might have shaped his difficult behaviours. In the second session Carl made it very clear that he was still troubled by memories of his childhood but had adopted the position that he did not want to think or talk about them anymore. We can also see in the extract the intense distress, sense of failure, exasperation and anger that adoptive parents can feel with a young person like Carl.

Anger and protest/vulnerability and protection

Attachment theory emphasises that the attachment system is dialectical. It simultaneously consists of the expression of vulnerability and the need for the provision of safety and comfort. However, at the same time it consists of anger and protest at why the attachment figures may have been temporarily unavailable, absent or slow to respond. As adults these two sides continue to co-exist. Hopefully, we develop ways of balancing the two feelings through an awareness of both feelings and reflection to help resolve the tensions between them.

One of our starting points for working in adoption and fostering contexts is a recognition that there are two sets of attachment needs that should be considered; that of the young person and also that of the adoptive parents and that the latter needs to express both sides of their attachment needs – protest/anger and vulnerability/safety, in the same way that the child does (see Figure 7.1).

Many therapeutic programmes for working with 'attachment-disordered' children stress the importance of dealing with children's anger as a priority, as anger is seen as getting in the way of new attachments developing (Hughes, 2007). A central premise in our work is that many adoptive parents and

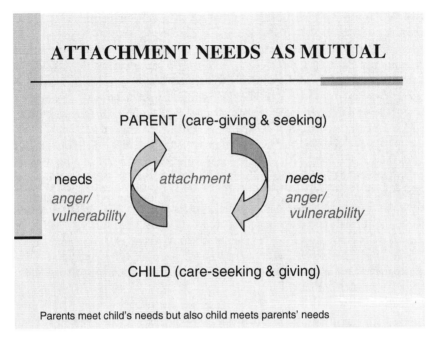

Figure 7.1 Joey's family tree

foster carers feel they have to suppress their angry feelings. Of course there are many reasons for this, not least the fear of re-producing the kind of angry relationships that the children may have previously experienced. There may also be a fear that things can escalate and that anger could get out of control so that a child needs to be removed. Interestingly, Carl remarked that although he recognised that he was at fault, and that his previous experiences shaped his actions, he did not want the focus of the sessions to be only about him. He accepted responsibility for acting badly, but also seemed to recognise that his parents needed help, in part because of what he 'had put them through' but we also felt that there was a more subjugated sense that perhaps they could also do things differently. This was captured by Brenda's response after our initial reflecting team conversation:

BRENDA: He needs me most, when I'm angry with him (tears), when I'm angry with him, when he's done something wrong and I'm shouting, that's when I should be able to go to him, tell him he's wanted, but I can't do it, and I don't know how to do it, and I know I should.
RD: So when you are angry with him, you see something hurting in him? Is it something like that?
BRENDA: No it isn't like that (inaudible/emotional) ... it feels like he doesn't care, so that's what I feel as his mum, instead of shouting. I should be saying, that you are still loved that you are still wanted. I don't know why

you are doing this but we love you. But I don't ... I say completely the opposite. I'm screaming at him, what are you doing this again for? I know it's not right ... but it's human nature. It's something I've got to work on. But we didn't speak for four days last week because he disappeared for nine hours. It's pathetic, I'm an adult but I was so angry. We just had a fantastic week away, came back and it was like he couldn't care less again. I know that's when he needs me most and I should be ...
RD: We can't be super-human and it's ok, more than ok, sometimes it's necessary to be a bit angry, to show that this is not ok. Do you agree with that Carl?
CARL: I'm not able to show my emotions sometimes, I'm like ... I don't blame her ... I deserve to be punished but I blank it, I cut off.

Here, Brenda poignantly illustrates the mixed emotions she felt in response to Carl's behaviours. Central to this is her sense of failure that she responds with anger to Carl just at the point where he possibly needed her most to accept him 'warts and all'. However, a potential dilemma for adoptive parents, as indicated by Brenda, is that because the child is seen as insecure and 'damaged' there is a pressure to suppress the expression of the anger as illegitimate – *'It's pathetic, I'm an adult but I was so angry'*. Such suppression is also explained by the fact that foster carers and adoptive parents may feel a pressure to act as 'professionals' and subject to potential criticism if they fall below acceptable standards. However, a most unfortunate consequence of this pressure to be 'perfect' can be that they come to feel that the only way out of the dilemma is to give up, and this sense of failure and wish to 'throw in the towel' can be experienced by both children and their parents.

Attachment narrative therapy

We have developed the broad framework of an attachment narrative therapy (ANT – Dallos, 2006) approach for work in the context of adoption and fostering. This approach consists of four stages:

Creating a secure base

This shares with other therapeutic modalities the creation of a sense of safety and security. A starting point is 'talking about talking' – checking with families what it is okay to talk about and exploring what they fear might happen should a conversation focus on the prohibited topic (Dallos, 2006). Using a reflecting team approach (Dallos and Draper, 2010) has also proved to be helpful with these families in gently allowing alternative explanations of their actions and negative feelings to be articulated. Normalising, using a developmental framework and locating difficulties in the family life cycle (Carter and McGoldrick, 1980) is helpful in moving away from a pathologising explanation for children's behaviour and the self-blaming position that can be taken by parents who feel they are failing and who can approach sessions with a defensive orientation. A central dilemma in this context may be the need to move away from an excessive focus on the child to the carer's own feelings and needs without creating an implicit message that they are therefore to blame or at fault. It is helpful to offer recognition of the difficulties they face and to validate their intentions and efforts. However, there is a delicate balance here between not subsequently retreating to an attribution of the problems as mainly in the child.

Exploration

Here the focus moves on to exploring beliefs, feelings and patterns of interactions. If formal measures of attachment are not available, questions from assessments, such as the AAI or the Separation Anxiety Test (SAT – Resnick, 1993) can be integrated into the therapeutic interview to help identify the attachment strategies being utilised by family members. Explorations, using genograms of transgenerational patterns of comfort and care-giving can also be helpful. We find that conversations about difficulties can be suffused with negative emotions and it is also helpful to initiate talk about families' hopes for changes over time and to look at when things have gone well as well as badly.

Considering alternatives

This stage utilises the material from the exploration stage and extends this to consider exceptions and unique outcomes. An important focus is on considering the parents' corrective and replicative scripts – what they have attempted to change and whether this has worked. Frequently, families here mention that they have wanted to be more emotionally available than their own parents had been but have experienced a sense of failure in not being able to achieve this. This can be linked to a consideration of 'unique outcomes' – times when their attempts have worked better or worse and then exploring how to build on and implement any experiences of success.

Maintaining changes and the therapeutic base

Having developed a sense of trust and support, it is important to discuss how support may continue in the future. This includes consideration of what problems are likely to surface in the future and what solutions they may adopt as well as sources of support the carers may be able to call on. Both children and carers may have experienced professional drift in and out of their lives, leaving them with a sense that people 'poke around' in their lives but do not stick around to offer reliable support.

The above offers a broad framework for the stages of the work and suggests a progression that is not simply linear. The focus on the secure base is consistent but as it is established, it is possible for the families to experiment and take risks in revealing their fears and vulnerabilities, as well as to accept their strengths.

Formats for exploration

We have developed a number of 'formats for exploration' that can provide a structure for discussions and explorations to promote reflection and change:

- Exploring working models – expectations, beliefs regarding self and other
- Exploring corrective and replicative Scripts
- Deconstructing attachment dilemmas – circularities
- Exploring discipline and attachment needs/contradictions
- Exploring comfort
- Exploring unresolved states – trauma and loss
- Sculpts to explore shifts in relationships

These formats are not exclusive and can often be employed jointly. However, they do allow points of focus and allow some clarity both for the therapist and also the family. A sense of the work being contained and focused can be helpful for all concerned given that there is often a considerable sense of chaos and overwhelming sense of everything going wrong.

Exploring working models – expectations, beliefs regarding self and other

A revealing activity can be to explore the child and carer's memories of the experience of the first day that they spent together as a family when their adopted children came to live with them. This obvious, but frequently overlooked exploration can be helping in prompting carers to understand that it can be a very different experience for the children than it had been for them. Verrier (1990) describes how adoption can be seen as an anxiety-provoking and even potentially trauma-inducing experience for the child – a 'primary wound'. The mix of experiences is all the more complex since as well as anxiety there may be reason to celebrate, the expectation of a new life for the child and the opportunity for infertile couples to become parents for example.

We asked Sue and Jonathon what they remembered about the day when their adopted children went to live with them and they told a story of how excited they had been. Sue, a head teacher at a primary school, had organised a treasure hunt in the house which took the children from room to room introducing them to their new home. Nichola (8) who, with her brother (6), had been living temporarily with a maternal aunt and her partner, said that they had cried all morning and the night before because they had not wanted to leave their current carer and family and would have liked to stay there. They had not wanted to show their upset to Sue and Jonathon. As well as being a good example of how capable children are at protecting their parents from upset, this gives us some insight into the different meaning that adoption can have for the children and parents. Sue was very surprised to hear the children had felt differently to her. She expected them to be a little anxious but had no idea they had been as distressed as they were by the move. In another case, Maria described how, on the day Sophie (8) had come to live with her, she had herself been distracted and upset as she had just learned that her Father had cancer. She had felt disempowered because there had been several professionals in the car with her as they collected Sophie from her foster carer to bring her home. Sophie had been crying and they had been comforting her. She remembered feeling excluded and when asked what she would have liked to have happened, she thought she should have been the one to comfort her daughter. It seems the seeds of her feeling she was unable to comfort or get close to Sophie may have been sown very early on in their relationship. Hearing the story of how her mum wanted to feel close to her at this time and understanding what had got in the way was helpful for Sophie who may have been wondering why her mum had been preoccupied and distant at the time.

Deconstructing attachment dilemmas

Our model stresses the importance of establishing a secure base and this is necessary for parents to feel safe enough to reveal the details of sequences of problems and the feelings and beliefs that maintain these. In the case of Mark and Brenda, a central part of this was helping them to feel safe enough to be able to express their protest and vulnerability without a sense of failure or shame. Brenda expressed clearly how she felt herself to be acting in a childish, immature way when she shouted at Carl and refused to speak to him for four days. She does not require parenting programmes to suggest to her that she could act in different ways. It seems clear that there is a conflict between what she knows to be the most appropriate ways of acting and how in the heat of the moment, she cannot stop herself reacting to Carl.

Exploration in detail of the sequence of such interactions is conducted to identify the feelings and underlying beliefs and expectations. It is possible to consider each step in the sequence of interaction and 'slow it down' and also to validate the feelings that family members are having. Most importantly, it is possible to understand this as a systemic process and to help remove the sense of failure that is fuelling both sides.

We heard for example that on the last occasion when things had gone dramatically wrong in the family, Brenda had voiced to Carl that at times the way he acted was as if he 'wanted it to be a family of three not four'. He took this as a veiled threat that Brenda and Mark wanted him to go, leaving just the three of them with his brother Pete. This led to Carl leaving the family home for days without letting his parents know where he was and

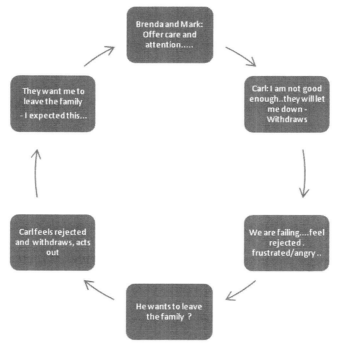

Figure 7.2 Repetitive pattern – circularity in Carl's adoptive family

reinforced their view that he didn't want to be with them. After hearing their recriminations on his return, he in fact rang social services and asked to be taken away which in turn convinced them further that he didn't want to be with them. Tracking these circularities and exploring the emotions, miscommunication and intentions embedded within them, is a core feature of our work in this context. It became clear that in the example of Carl staying out of contact for nine hours that he and Brenda both felt rejected by the other. When Brenda becomes angry, Carl interpreted this as proof that they really did not want him, as he had always suspected. Brenda likewise couldn't stop herself feeling that, despite all her efforts to show Carl love, his actions were communicating that he did not want to be in the family. In their interactions things happen quickly and these feelings and thoughts arise quickly without an ability to understand them or opportunity to alter the relational sequence of behaviours and feelings (see Figure 7.2).

Such mappings can form the basis for discussion with the family and the visual illustration can help to 'slow down' some of the heated emotions that are fuelling repetitive cycles of behaviours and feelings. In a family therapy session such sequences can be re-enacted (Minuchin, 1974; Dallos and Vetere, 2010) and with the help of the therapist and the team, examined in the moment in a calmer atmosphere, allowing the feelings that arise to be contained rather than escalating out of control. This experience of containment can help the family to insulate against repetition of the uncontained escalation when they return home.

In many cases the initial focus is on the child's behaviour and problems. Our work with Sophie (11) and her adopted mother Maria was requested when both individual work with Sophie and work with her mother by the post-adoption support worker was deemed to be unsuccessful and there were fears that the placement was at risk of breakdown and that Sophie would need to go back into care. During the course of the work, which also involved some formal assessment measures of attachment (AAI for Maria and The Story Stem for Sophie), we were contacted because Sophie had been suspended from her school breakfast club. This signalled a potential financial disaster because Maria was a lone parent and needed Sophie to be in the club so she could go to work. Things had been better between them since we had met with them several times and explored how their respective avoidant patterns could interlock so that there were periods of mutual avoidance and silence between them. In the meeting we discussed with Sophie, whilst Maria listened, details of the incident that had led to Sophie being suspended.

She described how she had been playing with a blanket which a boy came to take away from her. A tussle ensued and when the teacher intervened she was seen to unfairly blame Sophie for starting it. Sophie angrily threw a marble at the boy leading to the suspension. When we probed what Sophie was feeling and thinking at this moment in the sequence, she explained that it reminded her of how it had always been for her, that she got the blame and the rejection. Specifically it reminded her of how she had been the only one out of three siblings that was left in care by her parents and that she was 'not good enough':

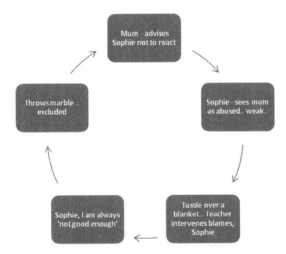

Figure 7.3 Circularity depicting Sophie and Maria's interaction

Maria commented at this point that she could empathise with how Sophie felt but still couldn't understand why Sophie did not see that behaving in this way would get her into even more trouble. At this point Sophie said she felt she had had enough of 'taking crap' from everyone. She also said that Maria had also let herself get walked over, for example by her previous partner (an emotionally abusive relationship) and should stand up for herself more. This prompted Maria to agree and say that as a child she had had strict parents and had tried hard to please people. This had led to her sometimes feeling weak and exploited. We remarked that there was a dilemma for both of them, between standing up for yourself and possibly getting into more trouble or walking away and feeling weak and rejected. When it was suggested that maybe there could be a third way – 'walk away to fight another day', Sophie considered this to be a good idea and immediately wrote it down.

In both these examples, it is possible to see that a shift of focus from exclusively being about the child, to an exploration of both sets of attachment needs is essential. Focusing on Sophie's behaviour is something that Maria had done extensively and she had typically instructed her about how 'not' to behave. Deconstructing an episode allowed some further understanding of why Sophie behaved that way but importantly about why Maria reacted as she did. Of course what is important in such analysis is that the parent does not feel criticised and disempowered. However, this does not necessarily occur and our experience is that the child is more likely to respect their parent as they see them becoming less emotionally reactive.

Exploring comfort: corrective and replicative scripts

The Adult Attachment Interview (George et al, 1983) includes questions about the giving and receiving of comfort when as a child the person was sick, hurt or upset. We have found that enquiring about how comfort is given and received and connecting this to trans-generational patterns of comfort giving is a useful area of enquiry for our work with adults and children who are struggling with intimacy/vulnerability and protest/anger. In the work with Sophie and Maria we observed that during our sessions, Sophie would often try to come closer to her mum in an attempt to seek affection and comfort. Maria appeared uncomfortable with this, and would flinch or withdraw in response to Sophie's approach. In her AAI Maria had described how there was little comfort for her as a child. She described how once when she had broken her leg, that she had been told to 'just get on with it' as it was 'only a broken leg'. In the same interview she also expressed the wish to 'do this differently' (corrective script) with her own children and felt disappointed that she ended up doing things in a similar way to her parents with Sophie. This mismatch between how she wanted to be and how she found herself behaving added to her sense of failure and she would respond in an angry and rejecting way towards Sophie because she was responsible for provoking this feeling. This exploration with both present enabled Sophie to realise that her mum intended things to be different, but because of her own experiences of receiving little comfort and affection, she had little to draw on in terms of resources as to how to do it differently.

We were asked to work with Nichola (8), and George (6) and their adoptive parents Sue and Jonathon when Children's Services became so concerned about Sue's parenting of the children that they were questioning if they could support the parents' application for an adoption order. They considered Sue's responses and disciplining of Nichola to be 'over the top' and inappropriate. Unlike her brother who had settled well and was described by Sue as affectionate and well behaved, Nichola was described as extremely self-reliant, controlling and disobedient. When physically hurt she would not show pain or accept comfort but, surprisingly, she would sometimes make a big fuss over little things, like a small scratch on her finger. An exploration of comfort giving and receiving again provoked Sue to reveal how she had wanted to be warmer and more responsive to her children than her own mother had been with her. Nichola on the other hand, because of her own experiences of severe neglect and of comfort being inconsistently available, had become self-reliant and appeared reluctant to expect affection and comfort lest she should be let down and find it not there when she needed it. As we discussed this with the parents we came to develop with them another understanding regarding comforting – perhaps Nichola was in some ways testing the water by seeking comfort when the stakes were low. Asking comfort regarding a small scratch on her finger involved less of a risk of feeling rejected than asking for care when she really needed it. We considered with them that if Sue was able to offer attention at these times, Nichola may be able to practise receiving it and become confident in its availability so that in time she might consider being comforted when she was really hurt or upset.

Exploring unresolved states – trauma and loss

In the examples so far the prevalence of unresolved states has been central. With Maria and Sophie we had the advantage of having undertaken formal attachment assessments and the AAI had identified that Maria's one significant romantic relationship, a man she had intended to marry, had been based on deceit. Her partner had in fact been married to someone else, had not told her about it and she found out through someone else. It is not surprising that a trigger point for Maria's anger and rejecting behaviour towards Sophie were incidents of deceit. Deconstructing what happened between them when each failed to meet the other's attachment needs unearthed this and enabled Sophie to understand why her mum may find her lying intolerable, and that it was not always just about her but about past hurts through betrayal. Gaining an understanding of unresolved states can indicate further how problematic sequences are maintained. In particular they may function to produce heightened emotional reactions to the child's behaviours leading to increasingly rigid applications of attempts at corrective scripts.

Exploring discipline and attachment needs/contradictions

On occasion, parental responses to children's behaviour can seem puzzling, bizarre or extreme. For example, at times Sue appeared to be particularly harsh regarding relatively 'minor' misdemeanours regarding Nichola. It is important to distinguish and explore with parents the different domains of attachment and discipline that underpin family life (Hill et al, 2011). Both Maria and Sue were professionals working with children in different contexts, Maria worked with children who were physically disabled and Sue was a head teacher of an inner-city primary school. When Sue punished Nichola for a wrong doing by a very public shaming, albeit at home, children's services became very alarmed, particularly because there were some parallels between the punishment chosen and an abusive experience that Nichola had experienced in her family of origin. Exploring with her the different domains in which she might offer discipline and comfort helped her identify that she had in fact been reacting as a head teacher might rather than a mother. Schools need to ensure discipline and order and this is a key priority for them to function and keep children safe. However, it is also a common assumption in fostering and adoption contexts that carers have a belief that it is important for children from disorganised and chaotic lives to have order and clear boundaries in their lives. Though relevant, this drive towards the discipline domain can predominate and leave such children feeling unloved and criticised. Furthermore, many maltreated children have in fact tried very hard to conform, to be good and to be self-reliant in order to survive. What has been missing is comfort and the giving of affection in a consistent way.

A discussion of the balance between attachment needs and discipline can help clarify some of the issues and explore how to combine the two domains. A primary framework is that both discipline and attachment responses are required to keep children safe, as is consistency between the carers. Sue started to see that the school context had been shaping her strategies and became more aware also of how this was compounded by her own experiences of being parented as a child which had been lacking in affection. Recognising her own wish to be more affectionate, but also lacking confidence about how to do this, along with how she had therefore relied more on her experiences as a teacher, allowed her to achieve a better balance between the attachment and discipline domains.

Sculpts to explore shifts in relationships/triangulation

Sculpting is an action technique that we have found to be usefully employed when family members are particularly anxious or preoccupied and are finding it hard to maintain a reflective state. It offers an opportunity for all family members to view relationship from each other's perspective and provokes discussion about similarities and differences as well as elaborating on the family story known up to that point. We prefer to initiate mini-sculpts, using coins or stones rather than to move people around in the room and this also enables family members to include those that are not present, and in this particular working context, it can be useful to provide an opportunity for a child to bring into the room symbols to represent members of a child's family or origin or extended family members of the child's adoptive family as well as those from the professional system. Such sculpts with objects encourages calm reflection and integration, the cooling down of emotions in the family. However, a more experiential sculpt can also be done with family members as the objects and this can be used to focus on the feelings about triadic processes.

We may use sculpts to show shifts in relationships over time and to help identify what has made the difference or to demonstrate the strength of attachments between family members which may not have become evident through talking. We have found that it can be useful sometimes for substitute carers to see for example the number of relationships a child is having to manage. This is particularly evident with looked after children who are most likely still having significant contact with members of their biological family as well as needing to maintain relationships with numerous professionals who are involved in their corporate care, the 'family' of professionals. It is not unusual for a sculpt to identify a looked after/adopted child as being triangulated – that is caught between two others who are in a conflictual relationship, on many fronts; between biological parents and substitute carers, between biological parents and social workers, between foster-mum and foster-dad. We know that children who are 'caught in the middle' can suffer extreme distress and a sculpt can be useful in demonstrating this to other family members, by providing an opportunity for a child to express how they feel and for conflicts to be resolved and for relationships to shift as a result. In our experience, even though foster carers and adopters are told about the importance of maintaining the significance of the child's biological family, it is still particularly common for carers to have a sense that the child might be able to 'move on' if they are able to forget about their birth parents and become free from the painful memories they have about them. Children, however may feel confused and disloyal that they still care about their family of origin and may even hold on to a hope of living with them again, when their adoptive parents and carers have done so much for them and are clearly 'so much better as parents'. Various reactions to such dilemmas are possible: for the child: to denigrate their own parents, denigrate themselves and to denigrate the adoptive parents – 'they are not that brilliant and superior to my parents as they think they are'. We find that such feelings are often subjugated and potentially destructive if left unspoken for the child and the carers.

Discussion

In this chapter we have described a framework for working with children who live in permanent placements with substitute carers either through fostering or adoption. In the UK, it is becoming more difficult for families to access psychological help for themselves and their children because of cuts to core services. It is claimed that what resources are available need to be focused on the child and this can mean that services are prone to overlook the attachment needs of the carers which we consider to be vital if they are to provide an environment in which traumatised children can heal and recover through establishing a more secure relationship with them.

The ANT framework emphasises that children who have experienced neglect and abuse will provoke extreme anxiety for most carers. Their attachment strategies, which may not have been revealed through the assessment process, may be provoked and may mitigate against them being able to maintain empathy and providing sympathetic caring for the looked after or adopted child. For therapeutic intervention with such families the establishment of a safe and secure base is vital. This is promoted by the therapeutic team paying due attention to the emotional climate in the room and having the confidence to explore and reflect on feelings, both their own and those experienced by family members. In the first session with Carl and his family some strong feelings were provoked in the therapeutic team when the parents revealed their sadness and despair. Acknowledging these feelings as well as validating the family's attempts to find new solutions was assisted by this sharing of emotions in the room, which in turn helped to provoke some significant changes in the family's relationships. The primary purpose of this attention to emotions and the attachment needs of both the children and the carers, is to help contain and avoid escalation and dysregulation of these feelings. By providing the family with opportunities for feelings to be expressed but with different consequences in the 'holding' context of the therapeutic relationship, the family is able to gain an experience of mastery, to contain inevitable conflicts and avoid destructive escalations. It is often helpful to speak with families on meeting them for the first time about how feelings will be managed in the therapeutic context, that it is expected that people might get upset or angry and to explore different ways in which this might be managed collaboratively. This often usefully initiates a conversation about how people in the family like to be comforted.

In order for this to be successful, we have found it helpful to be able to identify the attachment strategies that family members utilise at times of stress. This can be accomplished through formal assessment but is also possible if a framework of questions designed to unearth this information is integrated into the clinical work. As a rule of thumb, persons employing avoidant strategies will benefit from having the emotional climate 'warmed up'. Techniques such as enactment and intensification (Dallos, 2006; Dallos and Vetere, 2009; Minuchin, 1974) may be useful here and those who present as preoccupied and aroused will benefit from more cognitive interventions that seek to cool down their arousal and encourage more reflective functioning, the use of genograms and mini-sculpts may be helpful in this context. It is important to acknowledge with these families that they are often managing many complex relationships: with professional systems, the birth family, schools and so on. There is ample potential for unhelpful triadic processes, not least between the child, carers and the birth parents. It is therefore very helpful to see the genogram as a working document to be updated as new information emerges in the therapeutic process and to keep the potential for triangulation in mind and on the agenda.

We have found it useful to acknowledge with families that it takes some considerable time for looked after children to establish trust and a belief that they are valued. Specific studies of how these children increase their security are still scarce. Use has been made of play-based assessments (Story Stems, Steele et al, 2003) of adopted children both at the start of their placement and at subsequent intervals, and identified that the shift in children's representations towards security is patchy and slow to develop. They have discovered that children show some changes in becoming more able to trust adults but that the intrusions of powerful negative feelings and sense of catastrophe appear to be resistant to change. We have found it helpful to share this research with carers as a way of reinforcing the need to be patient, both with the children and themselves. Celebrating small changes is helpful to this process and in promoting resilience.

At the time of writing, we are hopeful of the potentially positive influences in the UK of the Reclaiming Social Work Model (Goodman and Trowler, 2012). This stresses the importance of professional social work utilising conceptualisations from attachment and learning theory, within a systems approach. The model is intended to promote systemic thinking about how to intervene in family life at points of difficulty and distress and offers a move away from the risk adverse and reactive practice of removing so many children from their families into corporate care as well as advocating new ways of working with those children who enter the care system. It fits with our emphasis in this chapter of working collaboratively and effectively with families to prevent placement breakdown and to reduce the repetitive cycles of distress and failure for children and carers alike.

References

Bowlby, J. (1979). *The making and breaking of affectional bonds*. London: Tavistock.
——(1988). *A secure base*. New York: Basic Books.
Byng-Hall, J. (1995). *Rewriting family scripts: Improvisations and systems change*. New York: Guilford Press.
Carter, E., and McGoldrick, M. (1980). *The family life cycle: A framework for family therapy*. New York: Gardner Press.
Cassidy, J., and Shaver, P.R. (2010). (Eds.) *Handbook of attachment: Theory, research, and clinical applications*. New York: Guilford Press.

Crittenden, P.M. (2008). *Raising parents: Attachment, parenting, and child safety*. Collumpton, UK: Willan Publishers.
Dallos, R. (2006). *Attachment narrative therapy*. Milton Keynes: McGraw Hill.
Dallos, R., and Vetere, A. (2009) *Systemic therapy and attachment narratives: Applications across diverse settings*. London: Routledge.
Dallos, R., and Draper, R. (2010) *Introduction to family therapy*. Maidenhead: McGraw-Hill
Freyd, J., Hullette, A., and Fisher P. (2011). 'Dissociation in middle childhood among foster children with early maltreatment experiences'. *Child Abuse and Neglect*, 35(2): 123–126.
George, C., Kaplan, N., and Main, M. (1985). *The Berkeley Adult Attachment Interview*. Unpublished protocol. Dept. of Psychology, University of California, Berkeley, CA.
Goodman, S., and Trowler, I. (2012). *Social work reclaimed*. London: Jessica Kingsley.
Hill, J., Wren, B., Alderton, J., Burck, C., Kennedy, E., Senior, R., Aslam, N., and Broyden, N. (2011). 'The application of a domains-based analysis to family processes: implications for assessment and therapy'. *Journal of Family Therapy*, Published online: DOI: 10.1111/j.1467-6427.2011.00568.x
Hughes, D. (2007). *Attachment focused family therapy*. New York: Norton.
Minuchin, S. (1974). *Families and family therapy*. Cambridge, MA: Harvard University Press.
Resnick, G. (1993). *Measuring attachment in early adolescence: A manual for the administration, coding and interpretation of the separation anxiety test for 11 year olds*. Rockville, MD: Westat Inc.
Steele, K., Hodges, J., Kaniuk, J., Hillman, S., and Henderson, K. (2003). 'Attachment representations and adoption: associations between maternal states of mind and emotion narratives in previously maltreated children'. *Journal of Child Psychotherapy*, 29(2): 187–205.
Tarren-Sweeney, M. (2010). 'It's time to re-think mental health services for children in care, and those adopted from care'. *Clinical Child Psychology and Psychiatry*, 15(4): 613–627.
——(2008). 'The mental health of children in out-of-home care'. *Current Opinion in Psychiatry*, 21: 345–349.
Trevarthen, C., and Aitken, J. (2001). 'Infant inter-subjectivity: Research, theory and clinical applications'. *Journal of Child Psychology and Psychiatry*, 42: 3–48.
Van Ijzedoorn, M.H., Goldberg, S., Kroonberg, P.M., and Frenkel, O.J. (1992). 'The relative effects of maternal and child problems on the quality of attachment: A meta-analysis of attachment in clinical samples'. *Child Development*, 63: 840–858.
Verrier, N. (1993). *The primal wound*. Gateway Press: Lafayette, CA.

Part III
Designing specialised mental health services for children in care, and those adopted from care

8 Ten years later

The experience of a CAMHS service for children in care

Megan Chambers

Summary

Emotional and behavioural difficulties experienced by children and adolescents in out of home care ('looked after children') play a major role in disrupting the stable placements, reparative relationships and opportunities for competence which contribute to better outcomes. Child and adolescent mental health services (CAMHS) are often asked to assist with these problems. Yet, delivering health care to these children is complex for many reasons, to do with the nature of the child protection systems, the range of issues presented by the children and the structure of many CAMHS. This chapter reviews the development of a specialist CAMHS operating in Western Sydney, Australia, over the past ten years. It describes a systemic approach to the work, both in terms of a shared care/shared responsibility model developed with the local child protection agencies and non-government care providers, and the implications of this for practice. It then describes the ways CAMHS processes need to be adjusted to allow for the special needs and circumstances of this population, and some clinical aspects of the work including issues for engagement, diagnosis and treatment. Particular dilemmas for staff in this service are also examined. These are all factors which need to be considered by clinicians approaching work with children and young people in OOHC, whether the context is a specialist service, a general CAMHS, or an individual practitioner.

Introduction

Children in out-of-home care face significant hazards in their dependent years. They have an increased rate of emotional, behavioural, social and developmental difficulties, in addition to an increased likelihood of academic delays and poorly treated speech and language problems (Tarren-Sweeney, 2008).

What constitutes effective therapeutic intervention, and how such interventions can be delivered are questions for many different services throughout the world (Simmonds, 2010; Vostanis, 2010). The choice of interventions and the framework for their delivery is influenced by theoretical assumptions about the nature of the children's problems, and their recovery and treatment: and by the complexities of services and service networks which include care and protection, therapeutic and educational elements in a variety of combinations (Leslie et al., 2005).

When a developmental psychopathology formulation is adopted, which postulates that the children's difficulties are the product of early abuse and neglect, attachment disruptions and ongoing developmental challenges, in the context of early biological vulnerability and acquired deficits (Cicchetti & Toth, 2009; Guttmann-Steinmetz & Crowell, 2006), then the interventions which are likely to assist them involve a coherent multifaceted and systemic response which includes the establishment of safe care, in the context of secure relationships, with opportunity for reparative developmental experiences and specific remedial opportunities (Golding, 2010; Leslie et al., 2005). Some of the indicators of better outcomes for this group e.g. stability of placements (Delfabbro & Barber, 2003), 'felt security' (Cashmore & Paxman, 2006), academic achievement and the experience of competence (Howard & Johnson, 2000), and connection with birth family (Maunders, Liddell, Liddell, & Green, 1999) appear to be consistent with this framework.

Mental health services can be overtly associated with facilitating many of these outcomes, when working with child protection systems. Placement breakdown and school failure are often due to behavioural and emotional problems (Aarons et al., 2010; Eggertsen, 2008). The emotional, behavioural and relational consequences of trauma and attachment disruptions effect the child and the carers (D'Andrea, Ford, Stolbach, Spinazzola, & van der Kolk, 2012; Dozier, Albus, Fisher, & Sepulveda, 2002; Fisher, Gunnar, Dozier, Bruce, & Pears, 2006) and contribute to the recurrent crises which disrupt the networks around the child and contribute to burn-out and dysfunction in the organisations concerned with them (Bloom, 2010). Yet there is an increasing knowledge base available of effective interventions e.g. to treat externalising behaviours and trauma-related symptoms, and facilitate relational recovery, improve affect regulation, develop effective parenting, and promote competence (Burns, 2003; Craven & Lee, 2006; Garland, Hawley, Brookman-Frazee, & Hurlburt, 2008).

How mental health services are best positioned to contribute to the child protection system is under discussion (Tarren-Sweeney, 2010). Variations include the degree of alignment to welfare services, and the level of specialisation required, either by individual clinicians or as a whole CAMHS team (Callaghan, Young, Pace, & Vostanis, 2004).

This chapter describes a child and adolescent mental health service specifically focused on working with children in out of home care, where the model of service delivery is integrated with the welfare services looking after the children, and with other therapeutic agencies and education providers. This systemic framework allows the team to influence case work decisions, respond to education concerns, to promote reparative parenting and to flexibly work with the child. The aim of this chapter is to articulate the implications of this focus, and the challenges of developing such a service. The benefits of a specialist service for this group are discussed.

Background

Many years ago, I worked as a consultant child and adolescent psychiatrist in a major children's hospital in Sydney. At that time, our 'on-call' duties involved calls to the Emergency Department for children and young people brought in by police and ambulance who were deemed to be 'out of control', or a risk to themselves or others. We would be called to see children who were distressed and angry, fighting all who approached them, abusing staff and needing to be 'contained' in locked rooms or sedated. Frequently they were found to be children in care, whose placements had broken down, who were currently homeless, and who were accompanied by adults who barely knew them. They would have with them no history or information, and they would have no health story readily obtainable. Staff dealing with these children in a busy hospital setting would be distressed, angry, dismissive, condemnatory, frustrated and confused. Why did these children need to arrive at Emergency? How had this become the pathway? What were emergency services supposed to achieve for the child? Most of these children were not 'mentally ill' – they were distressed and acutely dysfunctional, with major chronic problems exacerbated by acute situations. There had to be a better way for psychological and psychiatric help to be given.

Out of this frustration was born the idea of a service which could meet these children's needs more appropriately. It would be easy for welfare services to access. The team would have a level of expertise in the problems of young people with trauma and attachment disruptions. Staff in the service would be able to develop a relationship with, and knowledge of, the children and establish relationships with the service providers and welfare agencies. They would be able to act quickly and responsively to the early signs of crisis, and then move into non-crisis care. The service would operate within defined parameters to prevent overload, and unnecessary referral.

This service, the Alternate Care Clinic (ACC), has evolved over the past 10 years. Over that time, various 'lessons' have been learnt about ways to sustain and nurture functional partnerships and ways to adapt clinical processes for this client group (children, carers and services). These lessons are outlined here on the basis that the same dilemmas present to any mental health service or individual clinician engaged in this field.

The alternate care clinic today

The ACC is an out-patient mental health service for 'high needs' children and young people in out-of-home care (OOHC, referred to as 'looked after children' in the UK and Ireland) in New South Wales (NSW), Australia.

Statutory child protection and alternate care provision is administered in NSW by Community Services, a state government department. Community Services currently maintains the majority of kinship and foster placements in NSW, and also licenses a number of 'for profit' and charitable children's agencies (including indigenous children's agencies) to provide kinship and foster placements. These agencies are referred to as Non-Government Organisations, or NGOs.

The current ACC team consists of four health funded positions (psychiatrist, social worker and psychologists) and two psychologists employed within Community Services, who are seconded to the clinic for two years on rotation. There is a part-time neuropsychologist and a part-time clerical assistant. This staff complement has grown over time, by serendipitous increases in funding.

The service is located in Western Sydney, and is part of the CAMHS service for the area. Physically it has offices and therapy rooms within Redbank House, a tertiary referral in-patient and day-patient hospital. Western Sydney Area Health Service is defined by specific geographical boundaries and the ACC is limited to seeing young people who live within these boundaries. This area of Sydney, New South Wales, has a population of 1,200,000 people. It has a number of socio-economically disadvantaged areas, and high numbers of both refugee and indigenous families. The area has over 3000 children in predominantly kinship and foster care, and a number of small residential services for high needs children, run by NGOs.

The current form of the clinic evolved through discussions between the mental health services and Community Services in the local area. It is significant that these discussions were seen as joint problem-solving exercises – the problems of placement breakdown caused by the young person's behaviour, acute presentations and difficulty of access were the drivers on both sides. However, each service had different priorities – for health services, the acute presentations were a key clinical dilemma: for Community Services, the agenda of avoiding placement breakdown and achieving easier access to professional opinions and advice were high priorities. The service developed from middle-level management discussions (the leaders at a regional level in both services). Funding support was then obtained from senior management.

The service was developed for:

- *children and young people from 0 to 18 years* (deliberately all ages of young people under statutory care),
- *with a court order of two years or more* – to enable a capacity to focus on children in long-term care, as these were children for whom service provision was particularly poorly developed (children still in the child protection system were excluded, because of capacity issues),
- *who were in foster care, kinship care or residential care*, and,
- *who were classified by welfare services as having 'high needs'*. This defined a population of children of concern to Community Services, both because

of the difficulty and complexity of maintaining placements for these children, and because of the increased cost of support services for these children. These children are not necessarily the same group as health services would define as most in need of referral to a mental health service: nor the ones most likely to benefit from interventions. However (as in the discussion later in this chapter) there was a need to clearly define pathways to the clinic, and part of the partnership approach was to allow for the different priorities of the partners to be respected.

The ACC functions in significantly different ways to other parts of the CAMHS service. These differences are intentional and designed to meet the specific needs of this population. They include accepting referrals on the basis of severity of dysfunction rather than diagnosis, when there may have been no previous health involvement. Assessment is initially by senior and experienced staff. The intervention by the clinic is 'open-ended' i.e. there is no specific time frame or number of sessions. Cases are regarded as active (being assessed or in active treatment) or inactive (when nothing is required from the ACC). An inactive case can be re-activated as necessary at any stage until the young person is 18 years old and leaves the care of Community Services. This provision is to avoid the child being referred to new services every time there is a relapse or a problem develops (e.g. with change of placement, or change to high school). An ACC case is assumed to take more time than a usual community case, and case loads of clinicians are small.

Clinicians work with the child, their carers, the child's caseworkers, and their school, and with any other clinical staff involved. These people are held to represent the child's 'parent system'. *Mental health intervention is regarded as an integral part of the whole system's effort to stabilise the child and facilitate optimal development.*

The fundamental importance of partnerships

The ACC is embedded in a number of partnerships, both formal and informal. These partnerships are essential to the functioning of the clinic, and are continually evolving. There are three groups of partnerships – with other health services and providers, with public sector welfare services, and with the NGO care providers. Each of these groups is essential to timely and appropriate referrals, to successful and effective care planning, and to the delivery of therapeutic interventions.

Historical background – how the need for partnerships became clear

When the ACC was first envisioned, there was a long history of health and welfare sectors regarding each other as failing the needs of the children, and little sense of shared responsibility. Referral was often delayed and in crisis and accompanied by crises in care provision. Private health providers (individual counsellors and private psychiatrists) were sometimes involved, but there were recurrent issues around missed appointments, incapacity to respond to crises, and problems with the expense of these services.

Confusion about roles and processes was a regular complaint e.g. case decisions which therapeutic services regarded as significant to their work were often not discussed or communicated; working with foster parents was regarded as belonging to the province of the NGO rather than the therapist.

Resource issues also influenced the need for partnerships. Both Health and Community Services are stretched and any duplication a waste of resources.

These issues were identified in the early evolution of the clinic, and a framework established for both clinical case sharing and for problem resolution. However, it also became clear that the changing funding and policy framework, within which Community Services, NGO and health services exist, necessitated a regular management meeting structure so that changes occurring in any one service could be well communicated and impacts on other services modified. Over the last 10 years all agencies have seen major policy and resource shifts which have necessitated adjustments to the processes and policies of the clinic.

Partnerships with Community Services

The partnership with Community Services has four key objectives, operationalised as follows:

To facilitate timely and appropriate referrals. These referrals are generated within Community Services, supported by sufficient and appropriate information (defined by the clinic), and thoughtfully prioritised: and occur at a rate which the clinic staff can manage. They are discussed at a monthly referral meeting attended by both ACC and Community Services staff.

To facilitate joint ownership of difficult cases, and a commitment to shared care rather than shifting responsibility. Community Services staff remain engaged with cases referred to the clinic and commit to attending meetings/appointments and communicating regularly. The therapeutic agenda is seen as contributed to by all the adults involved with different aspects of the case rather than only by the therapist. Information flow is as open as possible. Personal relationships between the leadership of Community Services and the ACC/CAMHS services in the area have been important to develop over time, to sustain the partnership under pressure, for example a case eliciting publicity or political attention.

To facilitate mutual understanding of the child welfare and health systems to enable better partnerships to develop at all levels, and to decrease the chronic conflict between the systems which impacts on the children's access to care. There are several strategies related to this goal. A bimonthly senior management meeting reviews any issues arising in processes or specific cases, and discusses changes occurring in one or other agency. This group has also developed a range of flexible responses to urgent issues arising for either agency, for example advising about risk issues, making available urgent assessments, mediating with other agencies. This has significantly increased trust in the 'shared care/ shared responsibility' approach of the clinic. A third major contribution to this goal has been the commitment to the rotation of two Community Services psychologists to the staffing of the clinic. These are clinicians who have been working in Community Services advising case workers and managers, and who understand 'from the inside' the organisational thinking and priorities applied to cases. The two-year rotations give an opportunity for team members to work closely together, and share constraints and challenges arising in both sectors.

To promote increased knowledge of the psychosocial needs of the children and their carers within both welfare and health systems, to promote earlier referral and therapeutic case planning on a wider scale. Opportunities for case worker training, teaching for CAMHS staff, and specific consultations are used to increase the awareness of the psychosocial needs of the children. Over time, the ACC has tried to increase the referral of younger children, and has developed an open access policy to 0–5-year olds in care, to promote awareness of this 'invisible' group.

Partnerships with health services

The ACC works in the context of other CAMHS and paediatric services which may be involved with children and young people referred to the ACC. The ACC has the following goals in relation to other health services:

- To facilitate appropriate access to health care for children and young people in OOHC. This means promoting comprehensive assessment and treatment as necessary and appropriate.
- To avoid the duplication, repetition and fragmentation of health care of a young person.
- To avoid either over-diagnosis or under-diagnosis of a young person (Pecora, Jensen, Romanelli, Jackson, & Ortiz, 2009).
- To support health services (especially mental health services) in the delivery of timely health care to young people in OOHC.

The ACC works with other health services by offering consultations to, and shared care with other mental health services if requested, and ensuring that private practitioners are included in case planning and communication processes. Emergency departments are provided with management plans if a young person is likely to present, so that the information required is available (contact and medication details).

The ACC may be involved with facilitating service developments necessitated by resource or policy changes in one agency e.g. the policy that all children in care have a comprehensive assessment (including a developmentally appropriate psychosocial assessment) has created the opportunity to assist in the development of models and training of staff to use them. ACC staff give presentations to other health services to promote an understanding of the impact of abuse, neglect and attachment disruptions on children, and the implications of this for their carers.

Partnerships with NGOs

The NGO sector has increased in significance as the policy framework has changed in recent years, and this has necessitated increased clarity in a number of areas, including,

- Specific communication processes appropriate to the organisation of each NGO.
- Models for working with clinicians employed within an NGO, to avoid conflict, confusion and redundancy.
- Models for working with carers, and managing potential conflicts arising from tensions between the needs of the agency and the issues of the carers.
- The need to avoid an advocacy or mediation role between the NGO and Community Services e.g. over the need for more financial support for a child or the need to have more staff/smaller numbers of children because of mental health needs.

Partnerships form the structure to support our approach to the clinical work, by creating *access to the children and their carers, information about them and input into the case planning.* In turn, our clinical processes needed to be adapted to work in this context and with the particular challenges these cases represent. This is consistent with the experience of other mental health services (Landsverk, Burns, Stambaugh, & Reutz, 2009).

The adaptation of clinical processes

Referral processes

Children and young people are identified as in need of referral to the ACC by their Community Services case manager. This allows for direct involvement with Community Services, but introduces a range of biases, for example:

- Crises in placement become the major prompt for referral, and other problems are under-referred e.g. internalising problems, very young children for whom placements are easier to source (e.g. see Levitt (2009)).
- Services can assume that poor functioning is the norm, rather than an indication for intervention. Projections about 'badness' and hopelessness can play a role.

- Case managers and their supervisors vary in their sensitivity to and knowledge of the children, and in their enthusiasm for pursuing referral, sometimes because of capacity constraints. Children with no strong involvement from an adult are unlikely to be referred to any health service.
- There may be divided opinions about the need for referral, which effect engagement and treatment options later. The agenda of a referral could be to satisfy an internal welfare process, to save money by using a public sector service, or dissatisfaction with a current service provider.

Attempts have been made to increase the thoughtfulness of referrals and the knowledge base of case managers. These attempts include case manager training, to increase the awareness of the importance of early assessment and intervention, developmental and behavioural norms, and the nature of the referral process. Attempts are now underway to establish a case review process within Community Services, so that senior clinicians can be consulted on a regular basis to identify children at risk before the issue of breakdown dominates. Referral of children under five years-old has been encouraged.

Working in partnership has allowed the ACC to request significant information when a referral is made. Community Services commits to providing history related to abuse and neglect (including the notifications made about the child before coming into care), and the child's history in care. This is highly significant – the child who has lived in one family for most of their life will present different issues to the child who has had ten placements by the age of eight! In addition, information is supplied about any medical and psychological interventions, the educational history and an outline of the current relationship context, including access visits with family or previous carers.

Engagement

The ACC clinician aims to work with the child, the carers and the case manager, and must engage, and keep engaged, all three parts of the system. This approach facilitates a strong partnership, rapid problem-solving and a sense of mutual support. The aim is to increase confidence and sustainability and enable treatment to be implemented.

The older child or adolescent may have had previous experiences of assessment and treatment which have been unhelpful or even traumatising: or they may have lost a valued therapist or doctor. There may be many new adults in their life to be negotiated. They may resist even attending a meeting, and be humiliated by knowing people are talking about them.

Carers may have unrealistically high expectations of therapy. They may certainly view the problems as entirely the child's, and have no openness to being part of the process of treatment. They may be over-busy, especially if they have a number of young children in their care. They may be exhausted and isolated, with few resources to bring to working with the clinician, and resent the case manager who made the referral.

Case managers may be reluctant to include the ACC clinician in communications and decision-making. They may be overloaded, and want the case to simply go away. They may become anxious if carers are not happy, or if problems are raised in the assessment for which there is no easy answer.

All these issues need to be clarified at the beginning of contact with the ACC. The process of assessment, the reasons for it, what can reasonably be hoped for from it, and why different people are involved needs to be explicit. In particular, the approach to the carers and the case manager needs to be collaborative, respecting their expertise and commitment to and knowledge of the child. Carers are not the same as parents in usual community cases – they are closer to being other professionals intimately involved with the child, who need to work with the therapist if there is to be any chance of success.

The clinician must validate limitations, respect constraints rather than make demands, and give enough time and thoughtfulness to the process to become a helpful resource, and a source of stability rather than stress.

Assessment

The ACC has developed an assessment process which is similar to the usual CAMHS assessment, but has added elements.

1. The assessment begins with a review of the referral information, which may be quite extensive. *Much of the history which will be gathered will be in documents, rather than in the memories of the adults currently with the child.* This needs to be well understood – it is no good looking to gather a history from the carers or case manager, who will invariably have partial knowledge and confused stories about the child (some kinship carers may be the exception to this rule).
2. A 'worker's meeting' (a professional network meeting) is held, involving carers, Community Services, NGOs, school and therapeutic staff. If the child is in residential care, it is useful to have both direct care staff and their manager, and any clinician working with the programme. This meeting

    - Ensures the information about the child is current and complete.
    - Clarifies the system around the child, and assesses its coherence and the range of views of the child held by different adults. There may be conflicts already in the group e.g. between the carer and the school, or within the school group. Often it becomes clear that those present have not spoken to each other, and may not have been aware of each other's existence. The ACC works from the position that functional recovery for the child will involve all the components of the system around the child working together, to sustain the placement and the best possible care, sustain the school placement and recovery of academic progress, and to promote social skills and opportunities for competence, as well as

specific treatment. This meeting begins that process, and signals that model.
3 Appointments with the child and carers follow a usual CAMHS assessment model. The principal difference is the priority given to the framework of trauma, loss and change which impacts both the content and the process of the assessment, and a focus on the strength of the relationships between the child and their current carers. Questionnaires are particularly useful to cover the wide range of possible problems.
4 At this stage also a referral may be made to the neuropsychologist for assessment. This is particularly the case where issues of developmental delay and school failure require clarification, but also where executive functioning deficits are pronounced, ADHD has been diagnosed, and where communication difficulties have been previously identified.

Diagnosis

This group of children and young people have usually experienced a range of severe challenges in their early development. These are likely to have included perinatal drug abuse, maternal high stress, domestic violence, poor nutrition, direct abuse in many forms and neglect of their developmental needs. They are likely to have had disrupted attachments, which may have been of varying quality: and to have had traumatic experiences sufficient to create specific fearful memories.

These experiences will have contributed to the development of a range of psychopathologies, which are poorly encapsulated in our current diagnostic frameworks. The children are likely to have problems with:

- arousal, reactivity and the capacity to self-sooth, or problems with low arousal and discomfort when the situation is calm and predictable
- developing intimacy and trust in any relationships, leading to a range of reactions to carers and other children at home and at school. These can range from antagonistic and aggressive, to excessively compliant and fearful; withdrawn or 'clingy'; rejecting and oppositional; seductive and controlling; covertly stealing and spoiling – and a range of others
- affect dysregulation
- abnormal behaviours with food and eating, sleeping and toileting and bathing, dressing, self-care and sexualised behaviours
- deficits in school functioning, high impulsivity and distractibility
- decreased ability to play, both by themselves and with other children.

These difficulties (and others not listed) are likely to attract multiple diagnoses, such as Attention Deficit Hyperactivity Disorder, Attachment Disorder, Complex Trauma, Chronic Post traumatic Stress Disorder, Pervasive Developmental Disorder, Oppositional defiant Disorder, Conduct Disorder, Depression, Bipolar Disorder, Developmental delay.

There is a real sense that these diagnoses are clumsy ways of describing the complexity of the difficulties of the children, and run the risk of both over- and under-estimating their problems (D'Andrea, et al., 2012; Dejong, 2010). It is difficult to encapsulate the children's strengths and resilience, and acknowledge the effectiveness of strategies which may now look like symptoms, but which have been protective and effective at times in the child's life (Crittenden, Landini, & Claussen, 2001).

However, multiple diagnoses may help the adults around the child to 'see' difficulties in a number of areas rather than just one, e.g. conduct disorder. The diagnoses also influence the choice of treatment strategies, although the application of some evidenced based treatments to this group is complex (Chaffin, et al., 2006; Landsverk, et al., 2009; Newman & Mares, 2007; Zilberstein, 2006).

In addition the use of a multiaxial framework, with some acknowledgement of developmental stressors, and a measure of overall functioning can reinforce the complexity of the case. This may be of more importance as mental health services become funded on a case-based model.

Treatment

The approach to treatment represents the integration of a number of elements, which are used variably in different cases, based on the presenting problems of the child, the capacity of the carer to support treatment, resources available in the clinic, the age and developmental stage of the child, and their capacity to engage. These elements include:

- Individual, dyadic, and family therapies, focused on relationship building, increasing empathy and reflective capacity, and promoting attachment security.
- Problem-solving and skill-building sessions, both group and individual.
- Sessions focused on the young person's sense of self and clarity about their story, often involving members of their biological family.
- Medication reviews, when psychoactive medication is useful for clearly defined symptoms. There can be a need for medication to decrease arousal and reduce reactivity to assist in the acute settling of a distressed young person. This is in addition to usual uses of medication in this age group, and needs to be monitored carefully so that it does not replace other strategies for increasing safety and security for the child and their workers.
- Worker's meetings/email loops for communication and joint problem-solving.

The underlying therapeutic approaches used are based on trauma theory and treatment approaches, attachment theory and principles for building secure attachments, behaviour management strategies and family systems approaches (Arvidson, et al., 2011; Cohen & Mannarino, 2008; Lewis, 2011).

An overall therapeutic focus on the promotion of 'felt security' and the processing of traumatic events, organises the approach to crises in care and prioritises the experience of safety for the child, the carers and others working with the child- including the ACC clinician. Incidents are analysed in the light of the child's history of trauma and insecurity: re-establishing safety is seen as necessary to allowing proper reflection, problem-solving and skill building at all levels of the system. Changes in care arrangements, contact with birth family, developmental challenges are all approached with this focus. The OOHC world is often unsafe for children, in very many ways. Stability may not be attainable, they may be dependent on adults with little capacity to take care of them emotionally, they are often intimately living with other highly aroused and reactive children who may be intimidating, and they may have little opportunity to develop skills to manage themselves. Their lives may be disrupted and disorganised by events over which they have no control. This not only affects the child, but also the adults in their system – including the ACC clinician. It can be seen in the pressure for fragmentation, reactivity instead of thoughtfulness, the desire for instant solutions, the ever-present sense of neglect and deprivation, and powerlessness. This is perhaps the hardest therapeutic focus – yet the one probably most related to outcomes, given the strong positive effects long term of stability and 'felt security' and coherence (Cashmore & Paxman, 2006).

Several defined interventions are used in many cases by ACC clinicians, including:

The Reparative Parenting Programme, a nine-session fortnightly group programme developed by clinic staff. This programme teaches elements of trauma and attachment theory, reparative strategies, and behaviour management which ensures safety and strong connection. It also helps the carers look at their own responses and need for self-care. This programme contains elements from other parenting programmes, adapted for this group. It is currently being evaluated for wider use.

Family therapy, where a family group can be defined. Patterns of interactions that become problematic are defined and alternative patterns encouraged. Multiple factors influence the capacity of specific carers to build a reparative relationship with a particular child, to process traumatic memories, meet the child's needs for appropriate developmental experiences and build competence. Work with the biological family to facilitate their connection to the child may also be part of 'family work'.

Parent Child Interaction Therapy is used for some carer/younger child dyads, often in the context of other work.

Therapeutic work with this group is also influenced by other factors including the evolution of approaches to thinking about attachment-related disturbance, and the difficulties in their treatment (Minde, 2003; Newman & Mares, 2007), the increasing use of therapeutic models by foster care agencies and residential care providers which enhance the provision of trauma informed care (e.g. the ARC model, the Sanctuary model or the Neurosequential model of therapeutics) (Bloom, et al., 2003; Kinniburgh, Blaustein, & Spinazzola, 2005; Perry, 2009); and increasing clarity about specific evidenced-based interventions for children and adolescents, for example The California Evidence-Based Clearinghouse for Child Welfare (CEBC, 2012).

The treatment model used by the ACC is one of episodes of care. A treatment plan is established, and reviewed regularly. The case can be inactivated at any stage, but reactivated by the carers, the case manager or school concerns. The aim is to allow continuity of care, as needed, particularly as children negotiate developmental or accidental crises. The transition to high school and into early adolescence is often a time of heightened anxiety.

The staff team

The staff of the ACC has had to work through a number of challenges. Some were anticipated, and some have been unexpected. These challenges include:

The work is slow, and engagement difficult

There are lots of missed appointments. Those closest to the child might not see the appointments as important or as a priority. Many relationships may need to be negotiated for one case. The ACC clinician must become part of the communication flow, and facilitate this if it is not happening. *Outcomes are hard to measure* when the work is slow and multilayered. This can be frustrating and deskilling. Even basic outcomes such as placement stability may be difficult to evaluate, when placement disruption can occur because of carer personal reasons, or agency policy or funding changes.

Many CAMHS staff are not used to working in a systemic way

Their training is focused around individual interventions, which are specific, evidence based and designed to be delivered independent of context. With children in OOHC work must be done to allow the young person to use these interventions, and to allow their care context to support them in doing so. For example, many of the strategies of dialectical behaviour therapy are potentially useful to dysregulated adolescents, but until they feel safer and are settled in a care context they are unlikely to use them – or attend the appointments to learn them.

The staff must learn about the workings of the welfare system, and move away from a traditional health position of blaming the welfare system for the inadequacy of its provision

A genuine partnership in which blame is not the default position needs to be achieved, through understanding the different priorities, agendas and struggles of each department. People who have worked 'on both sides' (namely the seconded Community Services psychologists) find this easier.

Vicarious traumatisation is a recurrent risk

Of necessity, this work involves a detailed knowledge of the histories of our clients and the reality of years of abuse and neglect. It involves seeing the effects of this, and noticing their fears and powerlessness. Their carers may have similar stories, or may experience neglect from services and invalidation in their roles. Staying connected to these clients is likely to elicit frustration, anger, distress and an intense desire to blame the systems that allow children to be hurt and unprotected, and those that care for them to be abused.

Staff may have a significant struggle to assert their voice within the system around the child

If the clinician has no previous experience with the particular people involved, they must rely on their role in the ACC until their usefulness is felt by other parts of the system, and carefully define their goals and responsibilities, and be explicit in their communications. There are also occasions when the system around the child is under strain and does not want to hear about problems for which there is no solution. This can happen for example when the only placement available for the child is unsuitable and frightening: or when a decision is made to leave a child in a placement which is not really good enough, or when a child is moved because of the needs of another child. The toleration of outcomes which are not optimal for the child is distressing and difficult, and taxes the partnership capacity. It is necessary to validate these concerns and have a clear procedure for expressing them to the relevant managers. However, the acceptance that welfare staff are doing their best and often have the same concerns can lead to better dialogues over time, and closer relationships and greater capacity to input planning in the future.

There are many strategies which allow the staff to survive and even thrive in this work. These include:

- Regular supervision, both individual and external team supervision, which allows reflection on the emotional complexities of the work.
- A framework for professional record keeping and review of treatment planning which encourages articulation of goals and responsibilities in a case.
- Opportunities to develop programmes, to write, reflect and present on the work, and the particular aspects which interest individual staff members.
- All cases are allocated to two staff, which allows for sharing of decision-making.

- Thinking within a family systems framework is encouraged and used in supervision. This promotes thinking about emerging alliances, splits, blame, disconnection and over-involvement.
- Experienced clinical leadership to provide direction and anxiety containment during crises, and strong connections with partner agencies.

Discussion

There are many dilemmas in this work. There is a need to increase the sensitivity of case workers to the psychosocial needs of the children, and identify them as early as possible: yet the resources available to help the children and carers is small and the risk of overwhelming services that exist and exhausting staff remains high. A complex array of health and welfare personnel may be involved with resultant confusion and fragmentation, or carers and child may be isolated. Therapeutic staff may be in conflict with those making the case plan. Effective treatment may be available, but there may not be a context to support its implementation.

This chapter describes a model for a mental health service for children in OOHC. This model has strengths, based on its strong connections to other health services, welfare services and NGO care providers. This enables improved cohesion and support for interventions, and a focus on both increasing early referral (when help is more likely to be effective) and developing processes which maximise the effectiveness of all agents available. This integration of mental health services and welfare provision has been developed in other jurisdictions (Pecora et al., 2009; Tarren-Sweeney, 2010).

The ACC has adopted a model of recovery which prioritises maximising functioning, building stability and safety, working with carers and agencies to promote this and with schools to promote normalising functioning. The ACC staff see these aspects as fundamental to the success of other more direct therapeutic interventions which in turn should enhance the child's capacity to use real-life supports. The importance of using evidence-based interventions is clear (Landsverk et al., 2009), but implementation requires an effective framework.

Many components of this model are possible for other CAMHS services, provided staff are allowed to modify case loads and time frames, and are given support and supervision to work in a different structure. When the ACC works with other CAMHS services, missed appointments, complexity and communication difficulties have created the most frustration, for example establishing who to talk with about progress when it is not the person who brings the child to an appointment. Moving beyond mutual blame can also be an issue when time is short and anxiety is high, and the wider context unknown by either service.

The specialist team model has some other strengths. Specific strategies and programmes for this group can be developed. The plight of foster carers, and the challenges of working with them (and kinship carers) is particularly important – this is the group most proximal to the child, and most central to their recovery, yet often isolated, and unsure of their position between a worker and a family member. The group approach appears to be particularly successful. It can straddle the educational/therapy divide, and by normalising the difficulties experienced create both a capacity to raise particular issues frankly and allow the vulnerabilities of carers to come through, often with each other's support.

Of particular importance, and considerable difficulty, is the issue of establishing a common language and common goals of care with the range of services involved with the children and carers. These include case workers, carers, managers, school personnel and other health professionals. The ACC has a particular role in this, as it is positioned to be 'expert' within CAMHS, and can therefore assist in defining many of the children's difficulties in terms, for example, of attachment and trauma sequelae, rather than as major mental illness presentations. It can also assist in prioritising various aspects of case management which impact most directly on the child's stability e.g. decisions around birth family contact, and questions of placement change, and the need for accurate history. This is almost an advocacy role in the case management process, so that the therapeutic agenda is highlighted. Our regular partners are used to these issues being raised, and our support in pursuing them. Thus there is the potential for influencing the agenda in a wider range of cases.

The mental health/emotional and behavioural needs of children in care and the extent of these are established. The issue of meeting those needs and ways to assist recovery are much less clear. Our model promotes working with those closest to the child to enhance their capacity to be therapeutic for the child and build their recovery in their own context. Specialist clinicians are used for a mixture of direct and indirect work, but also have a brief to develop programmes and materials for other health staff (and welfare staff) to use. This is fundamentally a partnership approach where mental health services contribute to the expertise of others.

References

Aarons, G. A., James, S., Monn, A. R., Raghavan, R., Wells, R. S., & Leslie, L. K. (2010). 'Behavior problems and placement change in a national child welfare sample: A prospective study'. *Journal of the American Academy of Child and Adolescent Psychiatry*, 49(1), 70-80. doi: 10.1016/j.jaac.2009.09.005

Arvidson, J., Kinniburgh, K., Howard, K., Spinazzola, J., Strothers, H., Evans, M., et al. (2011). 'Treatment of complex trauma in young children: Developmental and cultural considerations in application of the ARC intervention model'. *Journal of Child & Adolescent Trauma*, 4(1), 34-51. doi: 10.1080/19361521.2011.545046

Bloom, S. (2010). 'Organizational stress as a barrier to trauma-informed service delivery'. In M. Becker & B. Levin (Eds.), *A Public Health Perspective on Women's Mental Health* (pp. 295–311). New York: Springer.

Bloom, S., Bennington-Davis, M., Farragher, B., McCorkle, D., Nice-Martini, K., & Wellbank, K. (2003). 'Multiple opportunities for creating sanctuary'. *Psychiatric Quarterly*, 74(2), 173–190. doi: 10.1023/a:1021359828022

Burns, B. J. (2003). 'Children and evidence-based practice'. *Psychiatric Clinics of North America*, 26(4), 955-+. doi: 10.1016/s0193-953x(03)00071-6

Callaghan, J., Young, B., Pace, F., & Vostanis, P. (2004). 'Evaluation of a new mental health service for looked after children'. *Clinical Child Psychology and Psychiatry*, 9(1), 130–148. doi: 10.1177/1359104504039177

Cashmore, J., & Paxman, M. (2006). 'Predicting after-care outcomes: The importance of 'felt' security'. *Child & Family Social Work*, 11(3), 232–241. doi: 10.1111/j.1365-2206.2006.00430.x

CEBC. (2012). *The California Evidence-Based Clearinghouse for Child Welfare* http://www.cebc4cw.org/ Retrieved September, 2012

Chaffin, M., Hanson, R., Saunders, B. E., Nichols, T., Barnett, D., Zeanah, C., et al. (2006). 'Report of the APSAC task force on attachment therapy, reactive attachment disorder, and attachment problems'. *Child Maltreatment*, 11(1), 76–89. doi: 10.1177/1077559505283699

Cicchetti, D., & Toth, S. L. (2009). 'The past achievements and future promises of developmental psychopathology: The coming of age of a discipline'. *Journal of Child Psychology and Psychiatry*, 50(1-2), 16–25. doi: 10.1111/j.1469-7610.2008.01979.x

Cohen, J. A., & Mannarino, A. P. (2008). 'Trauma-focused cognitive behavioural therapy for children and parents'. *Child and Adolescent Mental Health*, 13(4), 158–162. doi: 10.1111/j.1475-3588.2008.00502.x

Craven, P. A., & Lee, R. E. (2006). 'Therapeutic interventions for foster children: A systematic research synthesis'. *Research on Social Work Practice*, 16(3), 287–304. doi: 10.1177/1049731505284863

Crittenden, P., Landini, A., & Claussen, A. (2001). 'A dynamic-maturational approach to treatment of maltreated children'. In J. Hughes, J. Conoley & A. La Greca (Eds.), *Handbook of psychological services for children and adolescents* (pp. 373–398). Oxford: Oxford University Press.

D'Andrea, W., Ford, J., Stolbach, B., Spinazzola, J., & van der Kolk, B. A. (2012). 'Understanding interpersonal trauma in children: Why we need a developmentally appropriate trauma diagnosis'. *American Journal of Orthopsychiatry*, 82(2), 187–200. doi: 10.1111/j.1939-0025.2012.01154.x

Dejong, M. (2010). 'Some reflections on the use of psychiatric diagnosis in the looked after or "in care" child population'. *Clinical Child Psychology and Psychiatry*, 15(4), 589–599.

Delfabbro, P., & Barber, J. (2003). 'Before it's too late. Enhancing the early detection and prevention of long-term placement disruption'. *Children Australia*, 28(2), 14–18.

Dozier, M., Albus, K., Fisher, P. A., & Sepulveda, S. (2002). 'Interventions for foster parents: Implications for developmental theory'. *Development and Psychopathology*, 14(4), 843–860. doi: 10.1017/s095457940200409

Eggertsen, L. (2008). 'Primary factors related to multiple placements for children in out-of-home care'. *Child Welfare*, 87(6), 71–90.

Fisher, P. A., Gunnar, M. R., Dozier, M., Bruce, J., & Pears, K. C. (2006). 'Effects of therapeutic interventions for foster children on behavioral problems, caregiver attachment, and stress regulatory neural systems'. *Annals of the New York Academy of Sciences*, 1094(1), 215–225. doi: 10.1196/annals.1376.023

Garland, A. F., Hawley, K. M., Brookman-Frazee, L., & Hurlburt, M. S. (2008). 'Identifying common elements of evidence-based psychosocial treatments for children's disruptive behavior problems'. *Journal of the American Academy of Child and Adolescent Psychiatry*, 47(5), 505–514. doi: 10.1097/CHI.0b013e31816765c2

Golding, K. S. (2010). 'Multi-agency and specialist working to meet the mental health needs of children in care and adopted'. *Clinical Child Psychology and Psychiatry*, 15(4), 573–587.

Guttmann-Steinmetz, S., & Crowell, J. A. (2006). 'Attachment and externalizing disorders: A developmental psychopathology perspective'. *Journal of the American Academy of Child and Adolescent Psychiatry*, 45(4), 440–451. doi: 10.1097/01.chi.0000196422.42599.63

Howard, S., & Johnson, B. (2000). *An investigation of the role of resiliency-promoting factors in preventing adverse life outcomes during adolescence: A report to the Criminology Research Council of Australia*. Adelaide: University of South Australia.

Kinniburgh, K. J., Blaustein, M., & Spinazzola, J. (2005). 'Attachment, self-regulation, and competency'. *Psychiatric Annals*, 35(5), 424–430.

Landsverk, J. A., Burns, B. J., Stambaugh, L. F., & Reutz, J. A. R. (2009). 'Psychosocial interventions for children and adolescents in foster care: Review of research literature'. *Child Welfare*, 88(1), 49–69.

Leslie, L. K., Gordon, J. N., Lambros, K., Premji, K., Peoples, J., & Gist, K. (2005). 'Addressing the developmental and mental health needs of young children in foster care'. *Journal of Developmental and Behavioral Pediatrics*, 26(2), 140–151. doi: 10.1097/00004703-200504000-00011

Levitt, J. M. (2009). 'Identification of mental health service need among youth in child welfare'. *Child Welfare*, 88(1), 27–48.

Lewis, C. (2011). 'Providing therapy to children and families in foster care: A systemic-relational approach'. *Family Process*, 50(4), 436–452. doi: 10.1111/j.1545-5300.2011.01370.x

Maunders, D., Liddell, M., Liddell, M., & Green, S. (1999). *Young people leaving care and protection: a report to the National Youth Affairs Research Scheme*. Footscray, Victoria: Australian Clearinghouse for Youth Studies.

Minde, K. (2003). 'Attachment problems as a spectrum disorder: Implications for diagnosis and treatment'. *Attachment & Human Development*, 5(3), 289–296. doi: 10.1080/14616730310001596115

Newman, L., & Mares, S. (2007). 'Recent advances in the theories of and interventions with attachment disorders'. *Current Opinion in Psychiatry*, 20(4), 343–348. doi: 10.1097/YCO.0b013e3281bc0d08

Pecora, P. J., Jensen, P. S., Romanelli, L. H., Jackson, L. J., & Ortiz, A. (2009). 'Mental health services for children placed in foster care: An overview of current challenges'. *Child Welfare*, 88(1), 5–26.

Perry, B. D. (2009). 'Examining child maltreatment through a neurodevelopmental lens: Clinical applications of the neurosequential model of therapeutics'. *Journal of Loss & Trauma*, 14(4), 240–255. doi: 10.1080/15325020903004350

Simmonds, J. (2010). 'The making and breaking of relationships: Organizational and clinical questions in providing services for looked after children?'. *Clinical Child Psychology and Psychiatry*, 15(4), 601–612.

Tarren-Sweeney, M. (2008). 'The mental health of children in out-of-home care'. *Current Opinion in Psychiatry*, 21(4), 345–349. doi: 10.1097/YCO.0b013e2830321fa

——(2010). 'It's time to re-think mental health services for children in care, and those adopted from care'. *Clinical Child Psychology and Psychiatry*, 15(4), 613–626.

Vostanis, P. (2010). 'Mental health services for children in public care and other vulnerable groups: Implications for international collaboration'. *Clinical Child Psychology and Psychiatry*, 15(4), 555–571.

Zilberstein, K. (2006). 'Clarifying core characteristics of attachment disorders: A review of current research and theory'. *American Journal of Orthopsychiatry*, 76(1), 55–64. doi: 10.1037/0002-9432.76.1.55

9 Multi-agency and specialist working to meet the mental health needs of children in care and adopted[1]

Kim S. Golding

Summary

Many of the children and young people who are looked after in foster and residential care or are adopted have complex mental health needs that are not well met by traditional mental health services. These vulnerabilities stem from an interaction between pre- and post-care experience, and often include trauma, attachment and developmental difficulties. It is now widely recognised that these children are best served by dedicated services provided by professionals with expertise in meeting the needs of looked after and adopted children. This involves effective joint working between health, education and social care services and requires supportive policies and structures at all levels of the organisations. This paper will explore the strengths, challenges and barriers of multi-agency and specialist working to meet the needs of these vulnerable children and young people. This will be illustrated with case examples drawn from a multi-agency service in Worcestershire, UK.[2]

Introduction

Children and young people living in care are widely viewed as one of our most vulnerable groups. They are at high risk for a range of health difficulties, especially in relation to mental health. Ten per cent of children and young people within the general population in the UK will be diagnosed with a mental disorder (Green, McGinnity, Meltzer, Ford, & Goodman, 2005). Figures for children and young people living in care in England are much higher, approaching 50% for those living in foster care and rising to nearly 70% for those in residential care (Meltzer, Gatward, Corbin, Goodman, & Ford 2003). In addition 70–80% of children in care need specialist emotional or behavioural support (Skuse & Ward, 2003; Ward et al., 2008, in Sempik et al., 2008). Again, this need is most evident in young people living in residential settings (Stanley, Riordan, & Alaszewski, 2005). Such high levels of difficulties are not confined to the UK care system. A review of studies from Europe, North America and Australia confirms that children living in care have mental health problems approaching the level of clinic-referred populations (Tarren-Sweeney, 2008). Specific studies from around the world give a flavour of these difficulties. For example, 20% of children in care in Denmark have a psychiatric diagnosis and up to 48% rate as abnormal on the Strengths & Difficulties Questionnaire (Egelund & Lausten, 2009). In Australia, mental health problems have been found to be four times more likely within the care population (Milburn, Lynch, & Jackson, 2008), whilst in the USA mental health assessment studies have identified prevalence rates of 5–20% of young people in care with emotional disturbance. Higher rates are reported when developmental delay is also taken into account (Pecora, White, Jackson, & Wiggins, 2009).

Whilst the prevalence rates of mental health problems resemble clinical populations, the psychopathology of children in care is more complex. Tarren-Sweeney (2008), for example, lists the range of difficulties that characterise this group. He includes attachment and relationship difficulties, inappropriate sexual, food-related and self-injurious behaviours, trauma-related anxiety, and behavioural problems involving conduct, defiance, inattention and hyperactivity.

In the UK general population one-third of children and young people diagnosed with a mental health difficulty continue to have emotional difficulties and 43% of these have behavioural difficulties over a three-year period (Parry-Langdon, 2008). Given the continuing pressures of living in care, including placement instability and the lack of access to specialised services these figures are likely to be higher for children in care. Indeed a study by Broad (1999) explored the health of young care leavers and identified a high level of physical and mental health needs. A review of studies in the USA suggests that care leavers are likely to be at increased risk of mental health problems compared to those young people currently living in care (Pecora et al., 2009).

Children who have been adopted are less likely to feature on lists of vulnerable children (e.g., DCSF, 2008b). Although they have increased stability compared to many children living in care, children adopted from care have often experienced similar, if not more compromising, levels of adversity pre- and post-natally, as well as movement in and out of the care system. Adopted children and young people have complex identity issues to resolve (Gale, 2007). Additionally, families often adopt against a backdrop of failed fertility and loss, potentially leading to complex adjustment issues.

The increased mental health needs of children adopted from care compared to the general population have been recognised for many decades (e.g., Schecter, Carlson, Simmons, & Work, 1964). Although emotionally more secure than children living in foster care (Triseliotis, 2002), adopted children are still recognised as being at increased risk for psychiatric and behavioural difficulties (Barth & Miller, 2000). Children adopted later from care demonstrate difficulties in the short and long term (Rushton & Dance, 2006).

Reasons for high levels of mental health difficulties

The reasons for the high level of mental health difficulties in children living or moving from care are various and tend to focus on both pre- and post-care biological and social experience. Studies point to problems on entering care being compounded by care experience, leading to a complex interaction of past and present experiences (Jackson & Thomas, 1999; Mather, 2002; Milburn et al., 2008; Richards, Wood, & Ruiz-Calzada, 2006; Tarren-Sweeney, 2008; Ward, Jones, Lynch, & Skuse, 2002).

Prior to coming into care, disorganisation and high level of need within families frequently leads to neglect of health needs. Once in care frequent changes of placement, lack of advocacy and poor inter-agency communication can further hinder access to good-quality health care. In addition, low expectations and acceptance of bizarre or challenging behaviour by those directly involved with the children leads to under-use of mental health services, and a continuation of problems (Ward et al., 2002). I would argue that this is compounded by low expectations of service availability.

Developing integrated mental health services

Many authors have argued for dedicated mental health services for children in care, in recognition of their differing circumstances, and the need for effective inter-agency working for this specialist population. The increased risk of a range of health and education difficulties has focused attention on the importance of mental health, education and social care services working closely together at all levels (e.g., Arcelus, Bellerby, & Vostanis, 1999; Callaghan, Young, Pace, & Vostanis, 2004; McAuley & Davis, 2009; McAuley & Young, 2006).

Adopted children, with experience of neglect, trauma and loss are at increased risk of experiencing attachment and relationship difficulties (Gauthier, Fortin, & Jeliu, 2004), and mental health difficulties (Rushton, 2004). These difficulties can substantially impact both at home and school. Less has been written about developing services for adopted children, even though these children are also likely to benefit from multi-agency services with access to informed health practitioners who are willing to work closely with parents, education staff and adoption support teams.

Case example

Darren is a slightly built 6-year-old who has lived in foster care for the last three years whilst decisions are being made for his future. The current care plan is for adoption, but Darren continues to visit his grandmother and other relatives on a weekly basis whilst the court proceedings are brought to a conclusion. There is no current contact with Darren's birth mother whose whereabouts are not known. Darren's small stature and appealing looks give no outward clue to the confusion and rage he experiences within. He both demands and rejects care as he seeks to take control of his own safety. He is very attention-needing, not wanting his carers to leave his sight, and at times, and on his terms, he can be loving towards them. His relationship with his foster mother is however challenging. He is demanding and non-compliant, seeks her attention but returns affection with a pinch or bite. The carers remain committed to caring for Darren but acknowledge that they are becoming increasingly wary of him. They are also concerned that their 15-year-old daughter is spending more time at her friend's home as a response to the tense family atmosphere. Darren has been booked into several after-school clubs to try and relieve the pressure on the family, but school brings its own set of issues as Darren's difficulties spill over into his social relationships and behaviour in the classroom.

There are a range of questions facing the network supporting Darren which illustrate the complexity of supporting the emotional well-being of children in care:

- Where should the focus of intervention be? Does Darren need some form of direct therapeutic work to help him make sense of a life experience that is still not resolved? Should help and advice be given to the foster family in an effort to help Darren feel more settled with them? Or should attention be given to reducing the additional stresses that Darren might be experiencing, such as the intensive contact with some family members and lack of contact with others?
- What is the viability of the current placement? Is this placement meeting Darren's needs? Does he need more or less time spent within the family home? The team might even consider whether a different placement might be more suitable?
- What are the chances of securing an adoptive placement for Darren given the current behaviours he is displaying? How can potential adopters be given an accurate picture of Darren when he is currently experiencing such distress?
- How can school be supportive to Darren and meet his educational and social needs? Currently the risk of exclusion is high, which will only add to the pressures on placement. Can additional support be provided to the school to meet Darren's needs?

No single agency will be able to answer these questions or produce a plan which will provide Darren with the safety and security he needs. Working together, however, Darren's health, education and social needs can be considered holistically, and interventions put in place that might meet his need to feel safer, reducing his challenging behaviour and ultimately securing a more hopeful future for him.

Children living in non-biological families or residential settings can experience any of the mental health difficulties common to the general population. There is, however, increased risk of additional problems. These stem directly from early experience within the family of origin, the experience of separation and loss and the difficulties of adjusting to care by a substitute family or within a residential setting. These experiences place the children at increased risk of developmental, behavioural and emotional difficulties often within the context of attachment- and trauma-related difficulties, and leading to long-term problems in developing and maintaining relationships (e.g., Milburn et al., 2008). The challenge for the mental health practitioner is to maintain a holistic view of the difficulties, taking into account current and past experience. Deciding on a focus of intervention can be problematic. Difficulties might stem from past experience, current family functioning or problems more broadly within the social care system. The social care practitioner needs to maintain a similar holistic focus, with decisions about how far to seek help for the child, and/or carer, and when to attend to issues such as contact arrangements, suitability of placement, and legal proceedings. Education brings in another dimension as the children and young people are also coping with social and educational challenges. The importance of good communication and information sharing in the context of sound multi-agency working is obvious although often challenging to achieve.

Darren himself might have some ideas about how he can be supported. When YoungMinds asked children living in care in the UK about their perceptions and experiences of mental health stigma they found that these young people have some clear ideas about what they want from their education, placement and services including mental health services. The young people want to be listened to and understood. They want their carers and teachers to understand how to support mental health needs, reducing their need to engage with mental health services. When they do need a mental health service, they want mental health workers to take the time to build a relationship with them, including the use of creative engagement methods involving art, play, drama and music. The young people want to be involved in the design and delivery of mental health services, to make them more appealing and accessible. Children like Darren have experiences that make them more vulnerable to difficulties; it is therefore important that we take the time to listen to what they want. When we do listen we will notice that relationship is at the heart of meeting these children's needs (YoungMinds, 2012).

Barriers to receiving appropriate mental health support

Traditional ways of working, referral patterns and mobility can all contribute to children not receiving appropriate mental health support. Integrated and specialist services need to grapple with these potential barriers if they are to offer children, young people and their substitute families meaningful support and interventions.

Lack of stability and parental advocacy combined with more complex needs means that children living outside their family of origin do less well with traditional models of mental health services. The dominance of a medical model can lead to a narrow service which responds to children and young people based upon a diagnosis and recommended treatment, but fails to understand the complexity of the difficulties being presented (Callaghan et al., 2004; Milburn et al., 2008). The additional need for multi-disciplinary preventative help by those with mental health expertise can also be overlooked (Street & Davies, 2002).

Children and young people in care are less easy to engage with services and less well supported by typical operational criteria (Vostanis, 2007). In a study exploring the views of young people in foster care and their carers the young people report that they are put off services because of a lack of information, transport difficulties and inconvenient appointment times. They also experienced therapists as not understanding their language and culture. Carers in this same study reported difficulties with waiting times, off-putting venues and the lack of home visits and support for themselves (Beck, 2006). CAMHS therefore can lack the flexibility, sensitivity and accessibility required to meet the needs of this group of young people (White, 2006). Barriers include difficulties common to all children such as long waiting times, and the stigma attached to attending mental health services. This latter can be compounded for children who have experienced parental mental illness, further adding to their worries about accessing services perceived as being for 'mad people' (Beck, 2006). In addition more care-specific difficulties can arise. For example, Blower Addo, Hodgson, Lamington and Towlson (2004) identify difficulties with care arrangements, such as not having residential staff available to bring the child to sessions.

A study of adoptive families found a slightly different range of barriers to accessing services. Mental health professionals were perceived as not recognising the extent of the parenting challenge presented. This led to concerns about feeling blamed for the child's continuing problems and a sense of failure. As a consequence, parents waited too long before requesting help (Rushton, 2004).

Referral patterns can also lead to difficulties in ensuring that services meet the mental health and emotional needs of the children and young people. For example, referral might be prompted by the level of difficulty the child presents or the needs of a system to contain these difficulties, rather than on an accurate assessment of the mental health needs of that child.

Externalising problems are probably identified by referrers more readily than internalising problems, but the reasons underlying these difficulties can be poorly understood (see Arcelus et al., 1999). In addition, anxiety problems can be overlooked, especially when children are overly compliant, deal with stress by excessive self-reliance, or display difficulties through very challenging behaviour.

From clinical experience I would suggest that children with hidden emotional distress are at particular risk of not being referred or picked up by services. These children typically have a relationship style that tends to hide their needs from view. Thus Schofield, Beek, Sargent and Thoburn (2000) identify 'closed book children', who have adapted to early adverse parenting environments through the use of excessive self-reliance. They also describe 'too good to be true children' whose compliant behaviours can make them rewarding children to care for, but perhaps without recognition of the cost in terms of emotional health (see Crittenden (2008) for discussion of the development of these patterns of relating). Inter-agency meetings where knowledge and understanding of a child is pooled can be a useful way of highlighting concerns which are not recognised by individual practitioners or carers (Golding, 2004). When agencies work together, and information and expertise is shared, more appropriate referrals and interventions are likely (Milburn et al., 2008).

The mobility of children within the care system is a well-recognised barrier to receiving timely interventions. Those children who move placement frequently are less likely to access mental health services (Beck, 2006; Callaghan et al., 2004; Street & Davies, 2002; Vostanis, 2007). Frequent movement of placement leads to difficulties in building trusting relationships (Beck, 2006; Vostanis, 2007). When a young person lacks a confiding relationship the difficulties experienced are less well understood. This can reduce the likelihood of appropriate support being sought (Beck, 2006). There are additional difficulties for children moving to live out of the borough or county. In the UK, for example, the lack of a nationally consistent referral system and mental health services means that referrals and interventions begun in one geographical area do not transfer easily to a new geographical area (Beck, 2006). Problems in accessing services can arise when children are moved to the bottom of waiting lists in the new geographical area irrespective of how far up a list they have previously moved. In addition, referrals can be lost or delayed and case notes not transferred with children in a timely manner (McAuley & Davis, 2009; McAuley & Young, 2006).

Case example

Becky was adopted when she was 6 years old following frequent moves between the care system and home. The experience of early neglect and a lack of consistent attachment figures meant that Becky struggled to relate to her new family. From an early stage she displayed highly controlling behaviours that the family found difficult to understand or deal with. When Becky was 9 years old they sought help and Becky's name was placed on the waiting list for the local CAMHS. Whilst waiting for this support the family decided that they could no longer care for Becky and she moved to an emergency foster placement at the other side of the county, two more foster placements followed, and Becky's name was moved onto the waiting list for a different CAMHS team. Becky was 11 years old at the time of assessment by this team. The foster carers were finding Becky difficult to like or to manage. They found her controlling behaviours impacted on them and the other children they cared for. Becky had begun absconding from the placement and there were also some concerns about sexualised behaviour towards the younger children in placement. They were considering providing "28 days notice" on her placement. A professionals meeting was called and it was decided that a specialist residential placement would be sought for Becky. This residential placement lasted 18 months, during which time Becky met regularly with a therapist. It was difficult for the social worker to determine what this therapy consisted of as no report was ever provided. This, coupled with concerns about the quality of the residential provision and the escalating costs of this care, led to a decision to bring Becky back into county to one of the local Children's Homes. At nearly 14 years of age Becky's name was placed back on the waiting list of the original CAMHS team.

Becky's story illustrates the difficulty that young people can have in accessing appropriate mental health services when their mobility is high. Becky was 15 years old before being referred to a multi-agency team able to offer the network mental health advice. Team members supported the staff to care for Becky, liaised with CAMHS and education and attended multi-agency meetings as well as providing some individual support. Becky's last few years in care were stable but she needed this kind of holistic, multi-agency support much earlier.

Multi-agency and specialist working for children in care or adopted

Joint working between health and social services has been an underpinning vision for services to vulnerable children in the UK for many years. An Audit Commission report in 1994 led to the Quality Protects initiative (DOH, 1998). More recently there has been a focus on multi-agency working involving health, education and social care joining together in Children's Trusts and working closely with voluntary services (e.g., DCSF, 2008a; DFES, 2005; DOH, 2004). Guidance focused on looked after children has a similar emphasis with an additional focus on the advantages of specialist services to support children living in care (e.g., British Psychological Society, 2004/2010; DOH, 2009).

Outside of the UK a focus on the need for specialist services is also evident in policy discussion about children living in care. For example Egelund and Lausten (2009) highlight the need for more expert mental health services in Denmark, whilst Pecora et al. (2009) argue for improved mental health services and foster care systems in the USA. They suggest that these need to take a holistic perspective based on careful screening and assessment leading to the provision of more therapeutic environments.

A range of authors have considered the potential advantages of multi-agency specialist services to meet the mental health needs of children in care

(Callaghan et al., 2004; McAuley & Young, 2006; Richards et al., 2006; Vostanis, 2007; Ward et al., 2002). These include improved communication and information sharing, interventions tailored to the specific and complex needs of the children, and interventions tailored to a holistic and comprehensive understanding of the child, carer and the wider system they exist within. Children's mental health is viewed as only one component of interrelated difficulties that also involve relationships, development and learning (Anderson, Vostanis, & Spencer, 2004; Vostanis, 2007). Meeting a range of difficulties that can occur concurrently is helped when services are co-ordinated, with multi-disciplinary training to facilitate effective joint working (Ward et al., 2002).

Meeting the mental health needs of children adopted from care is likely to be similar in many ways to those for children who remain in the looked after system. Whilst there is a less complicated care system around children who have been legally adopted into new families, there is likely to be a similar complexity of need. Within the UK the main impetus for the development of collaborative, specialist services for adopted children and their families comes from the Adoption and Children Act (DFES, 2002). This sets out an expectation of collaboration between mental health and children's services, although this is not mandatory. Hart and Luckock, (2004) suggest that such an approach to multi-agency working is incomplete. In their view it does not go far enough in involving adoptive families as part of the partnership (Hart & Luckock, 2004). These authors suggest communities of practice as a framework for bringing together social, health and education support.

Assessment within multi-agency working

Multi-agency assessment of need ensures good working together and appropriate use of mental health services. Holistic assessment which considers mental health in the context of development, relationships and emotional well-being, and observes the child at home, school and community is recommended (Tarren-Sweeney, 2008).

Rather than relying on appropriate referral by those working closely with the child, mental health practitioners can usefully be a part of the team involved in care planning. They would contribute to discussion and provide appropriate assessment in a timely manner, ensuring early identification of mental health needs. The Stargate Early Intervention Programme is an example of such an approach piloted in Australia. Assessment by a multi-disciplinary team facilitated early access to mental health support, alongside helping carers to understand the child and the relationship. This improved the stability of placement and informed the planning process (Milburn et al., 2008).

It is important however that resources don't get placed into assessment at the expense of intervention. A study in Scotland suggested that the children's difficulties were well recognised by carers and professionals without the need for additional mental health screening. These authors identify the main gap in service provision as being around interventions to help children and young people with persistent, disabling and hard to manage mental health difficulties (Blower et al., 2004).

Mental health and social care agencies and practitioners need to work together to ensure that an appropriate level of assessment informed by mental health practitioners experienced in understanding the needs of children in care is available, backed up by relevant and accessible intervention services. Carers and other professionals need training in the identification of mental health problems, whilst carers can be additionally helped to recognise when they might usefully seek specialist advice (McAuley & Young, 2006; White, 2006).

Intervention within multi-agency working

Integrated multi-agency teams need to provide services at sufficient intensity and early enough to prevent mental health problems persisting through childhood and into adulthood (McAuley & Davis, 2009; Quinton, Rushton, Dance, & Mayes, 1998). I would argue that dedicated multi-agency services also need to be adequately resourced to allow good partnership working, with time for liaison and communication. This is a delicate balancing act that is not always easy to get right.

Vostanis (2007) points out that services need to be adapted to local need, with designated sessions or teams depending upon the size of the children in care population. In addition, a tiered response to need involving training, consultation and specialist interventions is important (Callaghan et al., 2004).

Working with instability requires close working together across disciplines. Street and Davies (2002) point out the difficulties when CAMHS and Social Care professionals don't work together. The CAMHS professional becomes frustrated with the social care professional, who they perceive as blaming the child for problems that lie within the care system. The Social Care professional on the other hand becomes frustrated with a CAMHS service that appears not to want to intervene without more stability in the care environment. As each understands the other's perspective then more imaginative solutions can be found. This shared understanding will lead to improved decision-making and more timely interventions, supported by appropriate care and school placements. Carers themselves are an important but not always acknowledged part of the multi-disciplinary team supporting the child. The carers have expert understanding about the individual child, and can be an important 'agent of change' in improving the emotional well-being of the child (Delaney, 1998; Minnis & Del Priore, 2001).

The rationale for requiring placement stability, often asserted by CAMHS, need not therefore be a requirement for mental health interventions. Whilst it is difficult to provide successful intervention in the face of instability, it is equally difficult to achieve stability whilst mental health difficulties are unresolved (Callaghan et al., 2004). Creative and innovative solutions to this dilemma are needed. These can include direct work with the child; even the longer-term psychotherapeutic approaches are no longer viewed as only viable when the child is living within a long-term family (e.g., Hunter, 1993, 2001; Kenrick, Lindsey, & Tollemache, 2006). Kenrick et al. (2006) describe the use of psychotherapy to help the child 'develop a new relationship to that past. Then, less burdened he can begin to reach out to take advantage of new opportunities' (Kenrick et al., 2006, p. 80).

My clinical experience suggests that practitioners working in a context of placement instability will need to provide a broad range of mental health interventions, working with child, family and wider network as appropriate. Early interventions can be offered alongside highly specialist interventions (Minnis & Del Priore, 2001). Prevention is seen to be as important as intervention, encouraging resilience through relationship building, as well as reducing mental health difficulties (Street & Davies, 2002; White, 2006).

Street and Davies (2002) suggest a 'levels of operation' model for mental health services for children in care, combining psychiatric, psychological, social work and childcare perspectives. The authors suggest that a range of multi-disciplinary interventions are needed to support these levels: managing behaviour via parenting advice and support, with more intensive interventions reserved for more complex and entrenched difficulties; therapeutic parenting to help resolve attachment difficulties; and life story work, taking into account current contact issues, to provide a foundation for resilience and psychological growth.

Young people living in care and adopted comprise a vulnerable group who are at increased risk of severe and entrenched mental health difficulties. The nature of these difficulties means that it is more difficult to support the children in isolation from other developmental, social and educational needs. Vostanis (2007) suggests that single-agency responses to meeting the mental health needs of these young people are unlikely to be successful. Instead there is a need to adapt services, therapeutic frameworks and interventions in a way that helps the young people and their carers to access and engage with a range of interventions.

Example: model of multi-agency working, Worcestershire, UK

The author has been involved in the development and evaluation of a UK-based dedicated support service for looked after and adopted children. This is described here as one example of how the mental health needs of looked after and adopted children can be supported using a collaborative approach.

The Integrated Service for Looked After and Adopted Children (ISL) is a multi-agency, holistic service, jointly provided and managed by Health and Children's Services. ISL works in partnership with all relevant agencies and services to ensure that children living in care or with adoptive families gain maximum benefits from educational opportunities, positive health and well-being, community and leisure opportunities and positive, stable social care environments.

The service consists of education support teams providing flexible, rapid response support to prevent exclusion and/or to raise achievement. A further team provides carer support and promotes inter-agency working. The aim is to maximise placement stability through the provision of advice and guidance about the mental health and emotional well-being needs of the children and young people.

Four health employees are seconded into ISL: two clinical psychologists, a community psychiatric nurse and the named nurse for looked after children. These professionals work closely with therapeutic social workers and education professionals to provide support to carers and the professional network surrounding the child. A range of mental-health-focused interventions complement the education-focused interventions of the education support teams.

At the core of the carer support team is a consultation service providing support to the carers/parents alongside their professional network. The goal is for a collaborative process with the dual aim of providing support and advice to carers and parents whilst facilitating inter-agency working (see Dent & Golding, 2006; Golding, 2004). Consultation is supported by a range of interventions including regular network meetings, ongoing advice and support and more intensive home-based interventions. There is an emphasis on supporting parenting to meet the attachment needs of the children and young people. This involves a small amount of assessment and direct work with children and young people alongside their carers; but ISL is seen as additional to CAMHS support rather than replacing it. Advice and support to a broad range of carers and parents is provided by training and group work with the aim of increasing understanding of child development and the attachment needs of the children and young people (see Golding, 2008; Golding & Picken, 2004). This is further supported by a range of training focused on the health and educational needs of the children and young people for carers and other professionals within the county.

ISL has been instrumental in the development of the 'Who Cares, We Care' children in care council, providing a voice to looked after children in Worcestershire. Additionally the nurse champions health assessment. She works alongside other colleagues to raise the awareness of the health needs of the looked after children and to implement The Healthy Care Programme (National Children's Bureau, 2005).

This brief description illustrates the breadth and depth possible when a range of professionals across disciplines and agencies are brought together to provide dedicated services to children living away from their biological families.

A range of research and audit-based evaluations has confirmed that ISL provides an effective additional level of support for the children, carers and professional network. This includes a pilot evaluation (Burgess & Smith, 2002) and an independent evaluation of service user views (McDonald, Burgess, & Smith, 2000). Group work programmes have been regularly evaluated highlighting high levels of satisfaction (Golding & Picken, 2004). Finally the consultation service has been the subject of a dissertation research project. Foster carers have a changed perception of the children and increased confidence and understanding following consultation (Golding, 2002, 2004).

Benefits, challenges and barriers

Whilst the benefits of multi-agency working are widely recognised challenges should not be underestimated. In this section I draw upon my experience within ISL, alongside the wisdom of other authors, to explore the benefits, challenges and barriers to providing multi-agency specialist services for children living in care and adopted.

Organisational policies can reduce the effectiveness of professionals working together if attention isn't given to policy, structure and process (Miller & Freeman, 2003). Multi-agency working can be undermined by lack of commitment to integrated practice at a strategic level across Education, Social Care and Health departments.

At its best, multi-agency working can contribute to the mental health of vulnerable children by facilitating working together across agencies and disciplines. More open lines of communication leads to a shared understanding of the children and young people and their mental health needs. In the process, practitioners gain a greater understanding of the roles of other agencies, improving access to and more appropriate referrals between services. This also reduces the likelihood that families will experience conflicting demands and advice as knowledge and expertise is enhanced across the agencies.

For this vision to be realised there are a range of challenges that need to be overcome. Bringing together agencies means bringing together different professional cultures, languages, roles and responsibilities, often against a backdrop of historical difficulties between those agencies. A genuine commitment to collaborative working will be needed if difference and difficulties are to be eliminated. In addition, practitioners are likely to experience unrealistic expectations of what they are able to achieve within existing resources, as integrated working is seen as the solution to everyone's problems. This can lead to heavy workloads and time pressures. Commitment from senior management will be an important part of creating a culture of both optimism and realism about what services might achieve.

A commitment to making integrated services and teams work requires a management structure that is prepared to give time to team and service development as well as ensuring that team members are getting the job done. Time is needed for building a team identity, shared vision and ethos and for reflection and the building of relationships. It is easy to give such tasks a lower priority in the face of high need, but ultimately without this, misunderstanding, and miscommunication will weaken service delivery.

Research has demonstrated that collaborative working at its best involves all team members, contributing to problem-solving and decision-making with a shared responsibility for actions. Team members share information and knowledge freely and have a good understanding of pooled and individual skills and knowledge within the team (Miller & Freeman, 2003). These authors also note that team working becomes ineffective when specialist skills become fragmented, inhibiting communication and the development of role understanding. Power structures and differences in beliefs about team working can further undermine team relationships.

A management system is needed that allows individuals within the service to meet the requirements of original agency as well as the new service. This means working with differing policies and procedures and finding some agreements between them. Attention needs to be given to what is effective information sharing and how to deal sensitively with issues of confidentiality and consent to intervention. Creative supervision and management processes for team members will support both working practice and professional development needs. Problems can arise when services are being driven by narrow targets and activity data without sufficient time for all these peripherals of multi-agency working. There also needs to be sufficient time for liaison, both at an individual case level but also between teams working within Health and Children's Services. This will have an impact on the caseload size of the individual practitioners tasked with the designated role of supporting the mental health of children in care and adopted.

Designated services are a helpful way of providing additional support to children and young people who have complex mental health and emotional well-being needs. These services can bring a specialised level of support targeted at the unique needs of the population. These services do however need to be embedded within core and universal services, allowing the children and young people access to the full range of support and interventions available to them. There can be a problem when a designated service is viewed as the answer to all the difficulties of the population leading to reluctance on the part of other services to accept referrals for these children. For example a local CAMHS team might view the designated service as removing a population of children and young people from their workload, thus giving them some welcome relief for their waiting lists. When the designated team is not able to meet all the mental health needs resentment can be felt on all sides. Understanding is needed to avoid such difficulties and allow each service to become a helpful resource for the other.

The impact of working with vulnerable and traumatised children on teams is also easy to underestimate, to the detriment of healthy multi-agency working. It is not unusual for splits, disagreements and even rivalries to develop both within and between services, leading to poor communication and conflicting decisions (Conway, 2009; Downes, 1992; Stott, 2006).

Conway suggests that such splits can be instrumental in placement breakdown, with a culture of blame developing between the services.

> ... in the system around the child there are two powerful dynamics at play: splitting, which divides the world and the people in it into separate, often hostile groups or states of mind; and projection, which fills people up with very powerful communications and feelings that can feel unbearable. In addition, there is a complex system around each looked after child that adds to the risk of these dynamics taking over, and can make working together feel like walking through an emotional minefield.
> (Conway, 2009, p. 23)

Opportunities are needed for professionals from across disciplines and agencies to meet for discussion and reflection. This can be supported by appropriate and independent specialists with good psychological understanding. This can lead to improved decision-making, reducing the potential for placement breakdown (Downes, 1992; Sprince, 2000, 2002; Stott, 2006).

Conclusion

Whilst the mental health needs of children living in care or in adoptive families are well documented, policies to meet the needs of such vulnerable children are less advanced (Wolpert, 2007). Multi-agency working and designated teams or posts are a way forward in meeting the complex and broad needs of this vulnerable group of children and young people. Bringing together health, education and social care agencies and encouraging partnership working between disciplines is not without its difficulties. A genuine commitment to collaborative working at all levels is essential. The time commitments involved in developing teams and services, providing and contributing to assessment and offering a broad range of interventions, training, advice and support should not be underestimated. If these teams and services are not fully resourced then multi-agency working becomes no more than rhetoric and children and young people are left once again falling between the gaps in services.

Notes

1 This chapter was previously published as: Golding, K. (2010). Multi-agency and specialist working to meet the mental health needs of children in care and adopted. *Clinical Child Psychology and Psychiatry*, 15(4), 573–587.
2 Case examples of children and young people are composite. Names and autobiographical details have been altered.

References

Anderson, L., Vostanis, P., & Spencer, N. (2004). 'The health needs of children aged 6–12 years in foster care'. *Adoption & Fostering*, 28(3), 31–40.

Arcelus, J. B., Bellerby, T., & Vostanis, P. (1999). 'A mental-health service for young people in the care of the local authority'. *Clinical Child Psychology and Psychiatry*, 4 (2), 233–245.

Audit Commission (1994). *Seen But Not Heard*. London: HMSO.

Barth, R. P., & Miller, J. M. (2000). 'Building effective post-adoption services: What is the empirical foundation'. *Family Relations*, 49(4), 447–456.

Beck, A. (2006). 'Addressing the mental health needs of looked after children who move placement frequently'. *Adoption & Fostering*, 30(2), 53–63.

Blower, A., Addo, A., Hodgson, J., Lamington, L., & Towlson, K. (2004). 'Mental health of "looked after" children: A needs assessment'. *Clinical Child Psychology and Psychiatry*, 9(1): 117–129.

British Psychological Society (BPS). (2004/updated 2010). *Briefing paper: Looked after children. Improving the psychological well-being of children in the care of the local authority.* Faculty for Children & Young People, DCP, British Psychological Society.

Broad, B. (1999). 'Improving the health of children and young people leaving care'. *Adoption & Fostering*, 23(1), 40–48.

Burgess, C., & Smith, K. (2002). *Supporting carers supporting looked after children: A description and evaluation of the work of an inter-agency project established in Worcestershire.* Unpublished document.

Callaghan, J., Young, B., Pace, F., & Vostanis, P. (2004). 'Evaluation of a new mental health service for looked after children'. *Clinical Child Psychology and Psychiatry*, 9(1), 130–148.

Conway, P. (2009). 'Falling between minds: The effects of unbearable experiences on multi-agency communication in the care system'. *Adoption & Fostering*, 33(1), 18–29.

Crittenden, P. M. (2008). *Raising parents: Attachment, parenting and child safety.* Devon: Willan Publishing.

DCSF (2008a). *Children's trusts statutory guidance on inter-agency cooperation to improve well-being of children, young people and their families.* London: DCSF.

——(2008b). *Children and young people in mind: The final report of the national CAMHS review.* Available at: http://www.dcsf.gov.uk/CAMHSreview/downloads/CAMHS-Review-Bookmark.pdf

Delaney, R. J. (1998). *Raising Cain. Caring for troubled youngsters/repairing our troubled system.* Bethany, OK: Wood 'N' Barnes Publishing.

Dent H. R., & Golding, K. S. (2006). 'Engaging the network: Consultation for looked after and adopted children'. In K. S. Golding, H. R. Dent, R. Nissim, & E. Stott (Eds.), *Thinking psychologically about children who are looked after and adopted: Space For reflection.* Chichester: John Wiley & Sons Ltd.

DFES (2002). *Adoption and Children Act.* London: TSO.

——(2005). *Statutory guidance on inter-agency cooperation to improve well-being of children: Children's trusts.* London: DFES.

DOH (1998). *The Quality Protects programme: Transforming children's services.* London: DOH.

——(2004). *National service framework for children, young people and families.* London: DOH.

——(2009). *Promoting the health and well being of looked after children: Revised statutory guidance.* London: DOH.

Downes, C. (1992). *Separation revisited: Adolescents in foster family care.* Farnham: Ashgate.

Egelund, T., & Lausten, M. (2009). 'Prevalence of mental health problems among children placed in out-of-home care in Denmark'. *Child & Family Social Work*, 14(2), 136–165.

Gale, F. (2007). 'Tackling the stigma of mental health in vulnerable children and young people'. In P. Vostanis (Ed.), *Mental health interventions and services for vulnerable children and young people*. London: Jessica Kingsley Publishers.

Gauthier, Y., Fortin, G., & Jeliu, G. (2004). 'Clinical application of attachment theory in permanency planning for children in foster care: The importance of continuity of care'. *Infant Mental Health Journal*, 25(4), 379–396.

Golding K. S. (2002). *Providing specialist psychological support to foster carers: The usefulness of consultation as a mechanism for providing support*. Dissertation submitted in partial fulfilment of the requirements for the degree of DClinPsy, Cardiff University.

Golding, K. (2004). 'Providing specialist psychological support to foster carers: A consultation model.' *Child & Adolescent Mental Health*, 9(2), 71–76.

Golding, K. S. (2008). *Nurturing attachments. Supporting children who are fostered or adopted*. London: Jessica Kingsley Publishers.

Golding, K., & Picken, W. (2004). 'Group work for foster carers caring for children with complex problems.' *Adoption & Fostering*, 28(1), 25–37.

Green, H., McGinnity, A., Meltzer, H., Ford, T., & Goodman, R. (2005). 'Mental health of children and young people in Great Britain, 2004. A survey by the Office for National Statistics'. Hampshire: Palgrave-Macmillan. In DCSF (2008b). *Children and young people in mind: the final report of the national CAMHS review*. http://www.dcsf.gov.uk/CAMHSreview/downloads/CAMHSReview-Bookmark.pdf

Hart, A. & Luckock, B. (2004). *Developing adoption support and therapy. New approaches for practice*. London/Philadelphia. Jessica Kingsley Publishers.

Hunter, M. (1993). 'The emotional needs of children in care: An overview of 30 cases.' *Association of Child Psychology and Psychiatry Review*, 15(5), 214–218.

——(2001). *Psychotherapy with young people in care*. Hove, East Sussex: Brunner-Routledge.

Jackson, S., & Thomas, N. (1999). *On the move again? What works in creating stability for looked after children*. Ilford: Barnardos.

Kenrick, J., Lindsey, C., & Tollemache, L. (2006). *Creating new families: Therapeutic approaches to fostering, adoption, and kinship care*. London: Karnac Books.

Mather, M. (2002). 'Securing health for children in the care of the state.' *Adoption & Fostering*, 26(4), 2–3.

McAuley, C., & Davis, T. (2009). 'Emotional well-being and mental health of looked after children in England.' *Child & Family Social Work*, 14(2), 147–155.

McAuley, C., & Young, C. (2006). 'The mental health of looked after children: Challenges for CAMHS provision.' *Journal of Social Work Practice*, 20(1), 91–103.

McDonald, P. S., Burgess, C., & Smith, K. (2003). 'Research note. A support team for foster carers: The views and perceptions of service users.' *British Journal of Social Work*, 33, 825–832.

Meltzer, H., Gatward, R., Corbin, T., Goodman, R., & Ford, T. (2003). *The mental health of young people looked after by local authorities in England*. London: The Stationary Office.

Milburn, N. L., Lynch, M., & Jackson, J. (2008). 'Early identification of mental health needs for children in care.' *Clinical Child Psychology and Psychiatry*, 13(1), 31–47.

Miller, C., & Freeman, M. (2003). 'Clinical teamwork: The impact of policy on collaborative practice'. In A. Leathard (Ed.), *Interprofessional collaboration: From policy to practice in health and social care*. Hove, Sussex: Brunner-Routledge.

Minnis, H., & Del Priore, C. (2001). 'Mental health services for looked after children: Implications from two studies'. *Adoption and Fostering*, 25, 27–38.

National Children's Bureau (2005). *Healthy Care Programme Handbook*. London: NCB.

Parry-Langdon (Ed.) (2008). 'Three years on: Survey of the development and emotional well-being of children and young people'. Cardiff: ONS. In DCSF (2008b) *Children and young people in mind: The final report of the national CAMHS review*. http://www.dcsf.gov.uk/CAMHSreview/downloads/CAMHSReview-Bookmark.pdf

Pecora, P. J., White, C. R., Jackson, L. J., & Wiggins, T. (2009). 'Mental health of current and former recipients of foster care: A review of recent studies in the USA.' *Child & Family Social Work*, 14(2), 132–146.

Quinton, D., Rushton, A., Dance, C., & Mayes, D. (1998). *Joining new families: A study of adoption and fostering in middle childhood*. Chichester: John Wiley & Sons Ltd

Richards, L., Wood, N., & Ruiz-Calzada, L. (2006). 'The mental health needs of looked after children in a local authority permanent placement team and the value of the Goodman SDQ.' *Fostering & Adoption*, 30(2), 43–52.

Rushton, A. (2004). 'A scoping and scanning review of research on the adoption of children placed from public care.' *Clinical Child Psychology and Psychiatry*, 9(1), 89–106.

Rushton, A., & Dance, C. (2006). 'The adoption of children from public care: A prospective study of outcome in adolescence'. *Journal of American Academy of Child and Adolescent Psychiatry*, 45(7), 877–883.

Schecter, M., Carlson, P. V., Simmons, J. Q., & Work, H. H. (1964). 'Emotional problems in the adoptee'. *Archives of General Psychiatry*, 10, 37–46.

Schofield, G., Beek, M., Sargent, K., & Thoburn, J. (2000). *Growing up in foster care*. London: BAAF.

Sempik, J., Ward, H., & Darker, I. (2008). 'Emotional and behavioural difficulties of young people at entry into care'. *Clinical Child Psychology and Psychiatry*, 13(2), 221–233.

Skuse, T., & Ward, H. (2003). *Outcomes for looked-after children: children's view of care and accommodation*. An interim draft report for the Department of Health.

Sprince, J. (2000). 'Towards an integrated network'. *Journal of Child Psychotherapy*, 26(3), 413–431.

——(2002). 'Developing containment: Psychoanalytic consultancy to a therapeutic community for traumatised children'. *Journal of Child Psychotherapy*, 28(2), 147–161.

Stanley, N., Riordan, D., & Alaszewski, H. (2005). 'The mental health of looked after children: Matching response to need'. *Health & Social Care in the Community*, 13(3), 239–248.

Stott, E. (2006). 'Holding it all together: Creating thinking networks'. In K. S. Golding, H. R. Dent, R. Nissim, & E. Stott (Eds.), *Thinking psychologically about children who are looked after and adopted: Space for reflection*. Chichester: John Wiley & Sons Ltd.

Street, E., & Davies, M. (2002). 'Constructing mental health services for looked after children'. *Adoption & Fostering*, 26(4), 65–75.

Tarren-Sweeney, M. (2008). 'The mental health of children in out-of-home care'. *Current Opinion in Psychiatry*, 21, 345–349.

Triseliotis, J. (2002). 'Long-term foster care or adoption? The evidence examined'. *Child and Family Social Work*, 7, 23–33

Vostanis, P. (Ed.) (2007). *Mental health interventions and services for vulnerable children and young people*. London: Jessica Kingsley Publishers.

Ward, H., Holmes, L., Soper, J., & Olsen, R. (2008). *Costs and consequences of placing children in care*. London: Jessica Kingsley Publishers.

Ward, H., Jones, H., Lynch, M., & Skuse, T. (2002). 'Issues concerning the health of looked after children'. *Adoption & Fostering*, 26(4), 8–18.

White, S. (2006). 'The mental health needs of looked after children'. In K. Dunnett, S. White, J. Butterfield, & I. Callowhill (Eds.), *Health of looked after children and young people*. Dorset: Russell House Publishing

Wolpert, M. (2007). 'Developing a policy framework for vulnerable children with mental health needs: Challenges and possibilities'. In P. Vostanis (Ed.), *Mental health interventions and services for vulnerable children and young people*. London: Jessica Kingsley Publishers.

YoungMinds (2012) *Improving the mental health of looked after young people: An exploration of mental health stigma*. London: YoungMinds.

10 Some reflections on the use of psychiatric diagnosis in the looked after or 'in care' child population[1]

Margaret DeJong

Summary

The current classification system, DSM-IV, inadequately captures the range and type of psychopathology seen in the 'in care' population of children. A combination of pre-natal influences, early interpersonal trauma involving the primary caregiving relationship, disturbed and disrupted attachment relationships and other significant losses and adverse environmental effects produce a complex constellation of symptoms and a pervasive impact on development that is difficult to categorise. The present chapter illustrates the challenges that DSM-V faces in conceptualising such complexity, highlighting unresolved topics such as quasi-autism, reactive attachment disorder and complex trauma.

Introduction

The run-up to the publication of the next version of the psychiatric diagnostic classification system (DSM-V) inevitably provokes a re-evaluation of our approach to diagnosis. A spate of recent articles (Angold & Costello, 2009) has reflected this, pointing out both the strengths and limitations of our current system. This chapter describes, from the perspective of a child psychiatrist working clinically with children who have suffered abuse and neglect, some of the difficulties that we encounter in our day-to-day practice in attempting to work within our current diagnostic framework. The focus here is on the severe end of a population of maltreated children; that is, children who have been in care, and are therefore amongst the most severely affected.

As a starting point, we might consider the purpose of a diagnostic system. One of its main aims is to provide a classification of diseases and disorders for the purposes of statistical analysis and epidemiological investigation. Another has been to facilitate research, in providing an agreed definition of conditions as a focus of study, which in turn has led to the development of an evidence base for treatment. A third aim is to provide an accurate description of a child's difficulties and a shared understanding in order to communicate effectively to different professionals involved in the child's care. Fourthly, it provides a rationale for treatment.

Two particular debates have featured with regularity in the psychiatric literature, both of which have posed problems for clinicians in this field. One is the categorical nature of our current diagnoses, which stands against the mounting research evidence that many diagnostic criteria are in fact more accurately described as dimensional; that is, characteristics relating to the diagnosis are continuously distributed in the normal population. The diagnosis in this case represents a demarcation based on severity, not on qualitative difference, which may contribute to uncertainty as to where the threshold lies.

The other major debate has been the vexed question of how co-morbidity is dealt with in the classification system. Many conditions, such as Hyperkinetic Syndrome and Conduct Disorder, or Anxiety and Depression, frequently co-exist. When is it more helpful to let them retain their distinct entities, and when is it more meaningful to combine them?

These debates are taking place against a background of vibrant research in fields such as neurobiology, genetics, and developmental psychopathology, which place a welcome focus on developmental pathways and processes, and push at the boundaries of our current, phenomenology-based classification system. How will it adapt?

Pre-natal influences

There is now growing research evidence pointing to an association between maternal stress during pregnancy and aspects of infant development (Bergman, Sarkar, O'Connor, Modi & Glover, 2007). As with all research on pre-natal influences there are methodological difficulties yet to be overcome (Swanson & Wadhwa, 2008; Thapar & Rutter, 2009) and the findings need to be interpreted with caution. Given the high prevalence of domestic violence in the population of parents whose children come into care, which is known to be exacerbated during pregnancy, it is an area of research with potentially important implications.

Substance abuse, like domestic violence, is highly prevalent in this population. Neurodevelopmental impairment resulting from substance abuse has been best documented in relation to alcohol. The well-recognised physical stigmata and cognitive deficits described as Foetal Alcohol Syndrome are likely to represent the extreme end of a spectrum of impairment; milder cases may not be identified. Research has also linked cocaine abuse in mothers with physiologic dysregulation at 13 months in infants (Schuetze, Eiden, & Danielewicz, 2009). However, clinical markers of substance abuse may be non-specific and especially in the absence of a clear history, not easily recognised.

Sub-threshold presentations

Sub-threshold presentations have become the subject of research interest (Pincus, McQueen, & Elinson, 2003). Follow-up over time has indicated that many such presentations tend to escalate into full-blown disorders (Shankman et al., 2009). There may be considerable functional impairment associated with a sub-threshold presentation, which is not given proper weight by the lack of a diagnosis. The problem is compounded by the fact that many of the psychiatric disorders that we see frequently in this population, such as Conduct Disorder, ADHD, PTSD, Depression and Anxiety are part of a co-morbid picture. It is often the case that a child may be sub-threshold on a number of different diagnoses; the resulting impairment is far greater than would be indicated by the diagnostic profile. If clinics are organised around diagnosis there is a danger that these children may not reach the threshold for treatment; an opportunity to reduce impairment and prevent further escalation may be lost.

Atypical presentations

Case example

A 14-year-old boy had been removed into care at 1 year old, having suffered extreme physical abuse. After an unsatisfactory kinship placement and a brief foster placement he was adopted at 2½. He was then a sad, 'depressed'-looking toddler who was difficult to soothe. He cried frequently, had nightmares, breath-holding attacks and violent tantrums. Eventually he settled into a stable adoptive family although the nightmares persisted until age 7.

By secondary school difficult peer relationships, provocative behaviour with aggressive outbursts and academic failure resulted in his placement in a very small private educational establishment. His academic struggles were puzzling given his average IQ until a neuropsychological assessment revealed marked difficulties in executive function. He was referred to child and adolescent mental health services at 14 because of some inappropriate sexual behaviour. His adoptive parents commented on his egocentricity, lack of empathy, poor understanding of emotional issues, and frequent apparently pointless lying around minor issues. The Autism Diagnostic Schedule (ADOS) revealed some autistic traits that did not reach threshold, but went some way towards explaining his problems in dealing with adolescent sexuality in an appropriate way. There was rather limited use of gesture and facial expression, although eye contact was normal. He demonstrated poor understanding of social context and reading of non-verbal cues, but could engage in reciprocal social interaction. He had marked problems in emotional processing which however could be assisted therapeutically, indicating more innate capacity than is seen in young people on the autistic spectrum. His self-esteem was very low, he was prone to feeling abandoned or rejected, he had poor emotional regulation and his mood was sometimes mildly depressed for brief intervals. He was beginning to get involved in drugs at the point of referral.

This case has features in common with many of the children we see who are placed in care after a background of abuse. The initial presentation at adoption suggests a traumatised young child although at the time of referral he does not meet the threshold for a diagnosis of PTSD. He had some mild attentional difficulties but did not meet the threshold for ADHD. He had traits, but was sub-threshold for a diagnosis on the autistic spectrum. His attachment security, as reported by parental history, seems to have moved from disorganised to insecure. He currently fulfils criteria for conduct disorder. Executive function, as is commonly the case in this population (Lansdown, Burnell, & Allen, 2007) is poor and contributes to academic underachievement. He is able to make friends easily but has difficulty sustaining relationships.

This young man is sub-threshold on a number of diagnoses, but only meets full criteria for conduct disorder. Conduct disorder by itself does not explain the extent of his impairment; he is significantly impaired on a cognitive, social, behavioural and emotional level. Nor does the diagnosis of conduct disorder point us in the most useful direction in terms of treatment. It is necessary to understand all of the implications of his early trauma and disrupted attachments to understand his current psychological presentation.

Nosological quandaries

The term *nosological orphan* was coined by Carlson (1998), referring to youth with severe mood dysregulation. The term seems particularly apt for the children and young people we see. Severe mood dysregulation (SMG) is certainly seen in the 'in care' population, where it continues to be difficult to classify in terms of diagnosis. The criteria, as adapted from Leibenluft, Charney, Towbin, Bhangoo and Pine (2003) and discussed by Baroni, Lunsford, Luckenbaugh, Towbin and Leibenluft (2009: 206–207), describe 'developmentally inappropriate increased reactivity to negative emotional stimuli at least three times per week, as well as sadness or anger most days, most of the time, noticeable to others'. Many foster carers would recognise this description. As the authors point out, impairment in SMG may be as severe as in Bipolar Disorder, which makes its absence in DSM-IV problematic.

Some clinical presentations that we see may be atypical of what is seen in routine psychiatric clinics, but attention is only now being directed at atypical forms of diagnoses, as being of interest in their own right. Clinical experience suggests that sub-threshold forms of autism or patterns of social disturbance that have autistic-like features may be seen quite frequently in this population although this has not been the subject of formal investigation. A post-institutional autistic-like syndrome has been identified in

Romanian adoptees (Hoksbergen, ter Laak, Rijk, van Dijkum, & Stoutjesdijk, 2005; Rutter et al., 1999). 'Quasi-autism' (Rutter et al., 2007) has atypical autistic features, including more flexibility in communication and a more marked, if abnormal, social approach, which in some cases resembles the disinhibited social behaviour seen in Reactive Attachment Disorder. There was found to be a trend for quasi-autistic symptoms to diminish over time with appropriate care in an adoptive placement, unlike the natural history of idiopathic autism. The possible relationship between autistic and attachment disorders remains unclear. Researchers within the autism field acknowledge that the broader phenotype requires further attention (Volkmar, State, & Klin, 2009). It will be important to investigate whether quasi-autistic presentations are also increased in children in care, with a background of non-institutional abuse and neglect (Rutter et al., 2007).

Some symptoms that we commonly see in children in care, such as sexualised behaviour, smearing faeces, or hoarding behaviour, do not point to a particular diagnosis, and may require a contextual understanding. For example, behaviour elicited in the context of a disturbed attachment pattern may not be observable at school. Sexual behaviour problems have been linked to both child sexual abuse and also to child maltreatment, family dysfunction or parenting deficits, and other developmental difficulties (Tarren-Sweeney, 2008). Tarren-Sweeney (2006) in a review of children in court-ordered foster or kinship care has similarly identified a significant number who display abnormal eating patterns according to carer report. A quarter ate excessively and 23 per cent gorged on food, while maintaining normal weight. Hiding or storing food (14%) and stealing food (18%) also occurred. These symptoms were found to correlate with maltreatment in care and specifically with maltreatment in the current placement. Other abnormal eating patterns, such as pica, were closely associated with developmental disability, and have been described in the learning disability literature. These patterns of abnormal eating are associated with other diagnosable psychopathology, but like the sexualised behaviour, do not fit a particular diagnostic category.

There are good reasons why the clinical presentations that we see may be different: our patients are subjected to a very particular kind of adversity that relates directly to the primary caregiving relationship, often occurs at a formative time in their development, and is likely to have very important neurobiological consequences (Glaser, 2000). This is frequently compounded by the more usual kinds of adversity seen across the spectrum of disorders: parental mental illness, socioeconomic disadvantage, drug and alcohol abuse and criminality. However, it is also characterised by highly unusual psychosocial experiences, such as removal from the care of biological parents, placement with alternative carers, and often, sadly, placement with multiple carers over time. Formulations of presenting problems need to consider prenatal influences and genetic vulnerability (although we have imprecise knowledge of these as yet), early infant development and attachment relationships, care giving experiences both within the biologic family and in alternative placements, as well as a range of psychosocial stressors. Complexity is therefore the hallmark of maltreated children, and they do not lend themselves to easy categorisation.

Social deficits

Children from a deprived background exhibit a whole range of social deficits that are inadequately described in the diagnostic classification system. Relationships are adversely affected by deficits in social cognition relating to the experience of abuse, such as a distorted attribution of hostility in others towards themselves. Wariness and lack of trust are common features, as well as a deep sense of shame and low self-esteem. Poorly developed social skills, and impaired ability to form relationships often occur, and may have a number of different causes. Attachment disorganisation and disorder may well be at the root of some of the social impairment, and have been described in relation to disinhibition or excessively controlling behaviour, but we have as yet to clarify what is attachment related and what is related to more general social development deficits (Green, 2003). Clinically a more fine-grained approach to assessment of social development is required (Byrne, 2003), and will help to advance our understanding.

Attachment

Some of the most illuminating research in this field has occurred in the area of attachment. Bowlby's (1969/82, 1973, 1980) conceptualisation of attachment followed by Ainsworth, Blehar, Waters and Wall's (1978) development of research tools to categorise it, has immeasurably improved our understanding of children's responses to caregivers, both within and outside of the care system. Nevertheless, many unclarified aspects remain, which have been well described elsewhere (Newman & Mares, 2007; Zilberstein, 2006). In particular, the concept of Reactive Attachment Disorder remains under-researched and of uncertain validity.

Reactive Attachment Disorder (RAD) has its origins in observations of institutionalised children, many of whom were unable to develop a selective attachment to a caregiver (Zeanah & Smyke, 2008). Both inhibited and disinhibited forms were described, although the latter has a more solid empirical and research basis. RAD is also seen in non-institutionalised children who have experienced maltreatment or severe neglect, and who have been subjected to numerous changes of foster placement at a formative age in terms of attachments with primary caregivers.

The diagnosis of RAD in a clinical setting poses certain difficulties. It is unusual, at least in western countries, to see the classical post-institutionalised picture, which encompasses severe deprivation effects including cognitive and developmental delays, stereotypic behaviour, and shallow, superficial social behaviour with comfort seeking from strangers. More often we see children who have some capacity to form attachments, albeit with a distorted and maladaptive pattern. Insecure and disorganised attachments are the norm in a population of maltreated children, the latter being reported in at least 65 per cent (Green & Goldwyn, 2002). At what point does a maladaptive attachment pattern, usually conceptualised as a risk factor, become a disorder? What, if any, is the relationship between categories of attachment patterns as delineated in research settings using research tools on normative populations, and RAD? In particular, what is the relationship between disorganised attachment and RAD?

Strength of attachment, as opposed to attachment security/insecurity, has been conceptualised in relation to institutionalised children, who may not have a discriminated attachment figure, or at best a weakly discriminated one. Findings of the Bucharest Early Intervention project (Zeanah, Smyke, & Settles, 2006) showed that only 3.2 per cent showed clearly recognised attachment patterns of security, as measured by the Strange Situation Protocol, compared to 100 per cent within the community group. Strength of attachment, or degree of differentiation, proved to be a more useful parameter in the institutionalised group.

One of the few studies to look at RAD within a maltreated sample (Zeanah et al., 2004) did consider the issue of degree of differentiation of attachment. They noted different patterns or subgroups of children in relation to degree of discriminated attachment and RAD, finding that symptoms of RAD could occur even where an attachment to a discriminated caregiver existed. This is in contradiction to the practice parameter for RAD set out by the American Academy (AACAP, 2005) which suggests that RAD describes children who have not developed a preferred attachment relationship (Prior & Glaser, 2006). Clearly further research is required within maltreated samples, looking at both strength of attachment as well as the pattern of attachment security.

Minde (2003) and others have asked whether attachment problems represent a continuum, with Attachment Disorder merging seamlessly into Disorganization and then into other forms of insecure attachment. Whereas a dimensional approach to assessing attachment insecurity may have advantages over a categorical approach (Fraley & Spieker, 2003), preliminary research does not suggest that the spectrum continues into attachment disorder. Minnis et al. (2009) using a questionnaire to measure RAD symptoms, reported that when used in a population of fostered infants and children, 30 per cent of those who fulfilled RAD criteria were rated on the Strange Situation protocol as securely attached. This raises a number of questions, including the possibility that RAD is not a purely attachment related phenomenon. More fundamentally, it raises questions about the validity of the concept and our attempts to measure it.

Other research findings have challenged the validity of the distinction between the disinhibited and inhibited form of RAD, which have been observed to co-occur in some children (Minnis et al., 2009). Rutter (2009) points to the fact that disinhibited attachment behaviour sometimes persisted in previously institutionalised Romanian orphans after they had been placed in satisfactory adoptive placements and were receiving good care, whereas inhibited attachment behaviour did not persist. Can one be confident therefore that RAD criteria are constructs of attachment-related behaviour, or might disinhibition be a more lasting social deficit resulting from extreme privation and its impact on social development?

The question of what is attachment-related and what is not is a familiar conundrum for the clinician. It is not just that the diagnostic boundaries of RAD are unclear; the existence of multiple co-morbidities can further confuse the picture. In popular usage, as seen on the internet, the concept of RAD has become very over inclusive, in danger of collecting symptoms and behaviours that are associated with deprivation and abuse, but have not found a comfortable home elsewhere in the classification system. In careful clinical practice, problems are appropriately classified as co-morbid conditions, such as Oppositional or Conduct Disorder, PTSD, ADHD or Anxiety Disorder.

In the face of such uncertainty a confident diagnosis of RAD is difficult. We are also faced with difficulties in obtaining an accurate clinical assessment of a child's attachment pattern, particularly in children over 5. Most research assessment tools of attachment do not translate easily into clinical settings. Furthermore, it is difficult to refine our assessment tools while there are such major and unresolved conceptual issues. As the criteria for RAD make explicit, they are not reliably applicable to children over the age of 5. Work that has been done to take a more fine-grained approach to describing clinically observed patterns of attachment (Zeanah, 1996) has been largely limited to infants and toddlers. Crittenden (1997) and others have developed systems of observation applicable to middle childhood, although a firm evidence base is lacking. Development is subject to a myriad of interacting influences; the older a child becomes the more difficult it is to disentangle an attachment pattern from other aspects of development.

Trauma

A response to the diagnostic constraints and dilemmas is well illustrated in one of the most important areas that we grapple with: Post-Traumatic Stress Disorder, and what is referred to in DSM-IV as 'Disorder of Extreme Stress Not Otherwise Specified' (DESNOS). There has been growing awareness of the limitations of the PTSD criteria, or indeed any cluster of apparently disconnected co-morbid disorders, to capture the range of symptoms and developmental impairment that results from the chronic, interpersonal trauma resulting from abuse by primary caregivers, described as 'complex trauma' (Cook et al., 2005; Herman, 1992). What one in fact sees is pervasive developmental impairment across all the domains, which is profound, enduring and difficult to treat. In an attempt to provide an inclusive and coherent diagnosis that accurately reflects this clinical reality, van der Kolk (2005) proposed the Developmental Trauma Disorder for inclusion in DSM-V. This proposed diagnosis suggests chronic interpersonal trauma as the primary stressor; dysregulation across many domains (emotional, cognitive, social) triggered by conscious and unconscious traumatic memories as its primary feature; and 'persistently altered attributions and expectancies' in terms of concept of self and others, as well as functional impairment in a number of domains.

Although there are controversies over the proposed diagnosis, the enthusiasm with which clinicians, including non-mental health professionals, have embraced the concept indicates a widespread perception of its usefulness in describing the clinical presentations that we see. A number of important characteristics of the proposal appeal to workers in the field. As in acute PTSD, and in direct opposition to most phenomenology-based diagnoses (Attachment Disorder being one of the exceptions), it makes a direct link to aetiology. In doing this, it crosses over a number of diagnostic boundaries and unites them under one conceptual framework. It also importantly emphasises the impact on development across many domains and provides a rationale for treatment approaches. The concept has spurred a number of innovative, developmentally based treatment programmes (Kinniburgh, Blaustein & Spinnazola, 2005).

One difficulty in relation to the proposed new diagnosis has been the relative paucity of data. The DSM-IV Field Trial included a retrospective study of 400 treatment-seeking traumatised young adults and adolescents (van der Kolk, Roth, Pelcovitz, Sunday, & Spinazzola, 2005), reporting a relationship between childhood trauma and disrupted development along the lines outlined by DESNOS. A recently reported analysis of four treatment studies involving a child sample ($N = 152$) and a sample of women with childhood maltreatment histories ($N = 582$) also shows a relationship between cumulative trauma and symptom complexity, with Complex PTSD in the adult group being most influenced by childhood, rather than adult interpersonal trauma (Cloitre et al. 2009). As the authors point out, further research is required to ascertain both the strength and specificity of a proposed childhood Developmental Trauma Disorder in terms of adult outcomes including Complex PTSD.

Professionals within the maltreatment field, although welcoming some aspects of the proposal including the emphasis on pervasive developmental impairment, may be concerned about a possible over-emphasis on trauma as an aetiological factor in maltreatment effects. Criteria such as 'Distrust of protective caretaker' or 'Loss of expectancy of protection by others' will inevitably raise questions about how much of the phenomenology is related to disturbances in attachment rather than trauma per se. Furthermore, there is relatively poor agreement as to what constitutes a traumatic experience. Neglect, for example, although very damaging to development, may not always be experienced as 'traumatic' in the conventional sense of the word.

Whether or not the proposal is successfully accepted into DSM-V, the term 'complex trauma' is now firmly embedded into clinical usage. This illustration of the divergence between clinical knowledge or practice and the diagnostic framework has been commented on in other fields such as eating disorders (Nunn, 2001). It is precisely this sort of tension that prevents the ossification of DSM, and propels us in new conceptual directions.

Impact on service provision

The constraints imposed by our current classification system, as applied to the maltreatment field, are not only a source of frustration for clinicians, they have an important impact on service provision. Too often Child and Adolescent Mental Health Services (CAMHS) are organised around diagnosis-led clinics, leading to fragmentation of service provision and dissatisfaction amongst users (Sturgess & Selwyn, 2007). Caregivers, whether looking after children in fostering, kinship care or adoptive placements sense that the difficulties the children experience are not adequately recognised and poorly described by the usual diagnoses, such as ADHD or conduct disorder. The treatment may be similarly narrowly focused. The experience of caregivers is therefore one of fragmentation and of being poorly understood.

The way forward

Big challenges face the maltreatment field, in order to improve the psychological support offered to children who end up in care. There is too large a gap between the known prevalence of abuse and neglect and our ability to recognise it (Gilbert et al., 2008). One way forward may be an increased emphasis on aetiology as well as phenomenology in the diagnostic assessment process. Increasingly, there are found to be links between psychiatric disorders and an experience of abuse, as illustrated in bipolar disorder (Garno, Goldberg, Ramirez, & Ritzler, 2005; Marchand, Wirth, & Simon, 2005). A better understanding of developmental pathways and careful formulation of individual cases will elucidate the link between early abuse and psychopathology, and hopefully lead to better recognition of a history of maltreatment.

A second challenge lies in trying to produce good quality clinical research in a field characterised by very complex presentations, with multiple, changing and interacting adversities. There have been inadequate research tools with which to describe the maltreated population, with an over-reliance on tools developed for ordinary clinic and community populations. The Assessment Checklist for Children (ACC) developed by Tarren-Sweeney (2007) is a great step forward in this regard, as it specifically includes symptoms observed in children in foster care. High-quality developmental psychology research has led the way in applying concepts such as attachment to various outcomes, and in developing our understanding of how this is linked to other developmental domains. It is now vital that this knowledge is joined to the expertise gained in clinical settings. How do we marry a developmental psychopathology perspective with our current diagnostic system? Perhaps by becoming less constrained by diagnosis, without forsaking it, in developing a range of observational schedules, semi-structured interviews and assessment protocols which provide a broadly based, thorough and developmentally sensitive clinical assessment, which is standardised to allow for research comparisons.

A third challenge is to improve multiagency communication around the needs of these children. Despite the known high prevalence of psychiatric disorder in children placed outside of their families (Ford, Vostanis, Meltzer, & Goodman, 2007), social workers and other front-line workers do not appear to acknowledge or recognise the presence of psychopathology in young children (Woodcock Ross, Hooper, Stenhouse, & Sheaff, 2009). If this is true, it has alarming implications which must be taken seriously. It reminds us of the role of diagnosis as a tool for communication with other professionals, and reinforces the impression that for non-mental health workers, the world of psychiatric diagnosis is obscure, specialist and remote from the reality of everyday work with maltreated children. In effect, the language of diagnosis constitutes a barrier to effective communication with workers who do not share our training. No one would consider that we should relinquish our diagnostic system, because it serves other purposes very well, but it does underline the importance of finding common language to communicate with our colleagues.

The difficulties outlined here in attempting to describe our patients in terms of the current diagnostic system are experienced in other fields as well. Genetic studies, neuro-imaging, and other biological approaches, as well as the field of developmental psychopathology are all contributing to an expansion of our horizons on the diagnostic front. The study of children in care as well as those adopted from care has much to gain from exploration in these areas; it will be fascinating to see how our diagnostic system adapts.

Note

1 This chapter was previously published as: DeJong, M. (2010). Some reflections on the use of psychiatric diagnosis in the looked after or 'in care' child population. *Clinical Child Psychology and Psychiatry*, 15(4), 589–599.

References

AACAP. (2005). 'Practice parameter for the assessment and treatment of children and adolescents with reactive attachment disorder of infancy and early childhood'. *Journal of the American Academy of Child and Adolescent Psychiatry*, 44, 1206–1218.

Ainsworth, M.D., Blehar, M.C., Waters, E., & Wall, S. (1978). *Patterns of attachment: A psychological study of the strange situation*. Hillsdale, NJ: Erlbaum Associates.

Angold, A., & Costello, E.J. (2009). 'Nosology and measurement in child and adolescent psychiatry'. *Journal of Child and Adolescent Psychology and Psychiatry*, 50, 9–15.

Baroni, A., Lunsford, J.R., Luckenbaugh, D.A., Towbin, K.E., & Leibenluft, E. (2009). 'Practitioner review: The assessment of bipolar disorder in children and adolescents'. *The Journal of Child Psychology and Psychiatry*, 50, 203–215.

Bergman, K., Sarkar, P., O'Connor, T.G., Modi, N., & Glover V. (2007). 'Maternal stress during pregnancy predicts cognitive ability and fearfulness in infancy'. *Journal of the American Academy of Child and Adolescent Psychiatry*, 46, 1454–1463.

Bowlby, J. (1969/82). *Attachment and loss, Volume 1: Attachment* (2nd ed.). New York: Basic Books.

——(1973). *Attachment and loss, Volume 2: Separation, anxiety and anger*. London: Hogarth Press.

——(1980). *Attachment and loss, Volume 3: Loss, sadness and depression*. London: Hogarth Press.

Byrne, J.G. (2003). 'Referral biases and diagnostic dilemmas'. *Attachment & Human Development*, 5, 249–252.

Carlson, G.A. (1998). 'Mania and ADHD: Comorbidity or confusion'. *Journal of Affective Disorders*, 51, 177–187.

Cloitre, M., Stolbach, B.C., Herman, J.L., van der Kolk, B., Pynoos, R., Wang, J., & Petkova, E. (2009). 'A developmental approach to Complex PTSD: Childhood and adult cumulative trauma as predictors of symptom complexity'. *Journal of Traumatic Stress*, 22, 399–408.

Cook, A., Spinazzola, J., Ford, J., Lanktree, C., Blaustein, M., Cloitre, M., et al. (2005). 'Complex trauma in children and adolescents'. *Psychiatric Annals*, 35, 390–398.

Crittenden, P.M. (1997). 'Towards an integrative theory of trauma: A dynamic-maturational approach'. In D. Cicchetti, & S.L. Toth (Eds.), *The Rochester Symposium on developmental psychopathology: Vol. 10. Risk, trauma and mental processes* (pp. 34–84). Rochester, NY: University of Rochester.

Ford, T., Vostanis, P., Meltzer, H., & Goodman, R. (2007). 'Psychiatric disorder among British children looked after by local authorities: Comparison with children living in private households'. *British Journal of Psychiatry*, 190, 319–325.

Fraley, R.C., & Spieker, S.T. (2003). 'Are infant attachment patterns continuously or categorically distributed? A taxometric analysis of Strange Situation behaviour'. *Developmental Psychology*, 39, 337–404.

Garno, J.L., Goldberg, J.F., Ramirez, P.M., & Ritzler, B.A. (2005). 'Impact of childhood abuse on the clinical course of bipolar disorder'. *The British Journal of Psychiatry*, 186, 121–125.

Gilbert, R., Kemp, A., Thoburn, J., Sidebotham, P., Radford, L., Glaser, D., et al. (2008) 'Recognising and responding to child maltreatment'. *The Lancet, December issue*, 21–34.

Glaser, D. (2000). 'Child abuse and neglect and the brain – a review'. *Journal of Child Psychology and Psychiatry*, 41, 97–116.

Green, J. (2003). 'Are attachment disorders best seen as social impairment syndromes?' *Attachment and Human Development*, 5, 259–264.

Green, J.M., & Goldwyn, R. (2002). 'Annotation: Attachment disorganisation and psychopathology: New findings in attachment research and their potential implications for developmental psychopathology in childhood'. *Journal of Child Psychology and Psychiatry*, 43, 835–846.

Herman, J. (1992). 'Complex PTSD: A syndrome in survivors of prolonged and repeated trauma'. *Journal of Traumatic Stress*, 5, 377–391.

Hoksbergen, R., ter Laak, J., Rijk, K., van Dijkum, C., & Stoutjesdijk, F. (2005). 'Post-institutional autistic syndrome in Romanian adoptees'. *Journal of Autism and Developmental Disorders*, 35, 615–623.

Kinniburgh, K.J., Blaustein, M., & Spinnazola, J. (2005). 'Attachment, self-regulation and competency'. *Psychiatric Annals*, 35, 424–430.

Lansdown, R., Burnell, A., & Allen, M. (2007). 'Is it that they won't do it, or is it that they can't? Executive functioning and children who have been fostered and adopted'. *Adoption & Fostering*, 31, 1–10

Leibenluft, E., Charney, D.S., Towbin, K.E., Bhangoo, R.K., & Pine, D.S. (2003). 'Defining clinical phenotypes of juvenile mania'. *American Journal of Psychiatry*, 160, 430–437.

Marchand, W.R., Wirth, B.S., & Simon, M.S.W.C. (2005). 'Adverse life events and pediatric bipolar disorder in a community mental health setting'. *Community Mental Health Journal*, 41, 67–75.

Minde, K. (2003). 'Attachment problems as a spectrum disorder: Implications for diagnosis and treatment'. *Attachment & Human Development*, 5, 289–296.

Minnis, H., Green, J., O'Connor, T.G., Liew, A., Glaser, D., Taylor, E., et al. (2009). 'An exploratory study of the association between reactive attachment disorder and attachment narratives in early school-age children'. *Journal of Child Psychiatry and Psychology*, 50, 931–942.

Newman, L., & Mares, S. (2007). 'Recent advances in the theories of and interventions with attachment disorders'. *Current Opinion in Psychiatry*, 20, 343–348.

Nunn, K. (2001). 'In search of new wineskins: The phenomenology of anorexia nervosa, not covered in DSM or ICD'. *Clinical Child Psychology and Psychiatry*, 6, 1359–1045.

Pincus, H. A., McQueen, L.E., & Elinson, L. (2003). 'Subthreshold mental disorders: Nosological and research recommendations'. In K.A. Phillips, M.B. First and H.A. Pincus (Eds.), *Advancing DSM: Dilemmas in psychiatric diagnosis* (pp. 129–144). Washington, DC: American Psychiatric Association.

Prior, V., & Glaser, D. (2006). *Understanding attachment and attachment disorders: Theory, evidence and practice*. London and Philadelphia: Jessica Kingsley Publishers.

Rutter, M. (2009). 'Emanuel Miller Lecture: Attachment insecurity, disinhibited attachment, and attachment disorders: Where do research findings leave the concepts?'. *Journal of Child Psychology and Psychiatry*, 50, 529–543.

Rutter, M., Anderson-Wood, L., Beckett, C., Bredenkamp, D., Castle, J., Groothus, C., (1999). 'Quasi-attachment patterns following severe early global privation'. *Journal of Child Psychology and Psychiatry*, 40, 537–549.

Rutter, M., Kreppner, J., Croft, C., Murin, M., Colvert, E., Beckett, C.,. (2007). 'Early adolescent outcomes of institutionally deprived and non-deprived adoptees. III. Quasi-autism'. *Journal of Child Psychology and Psychiatry*, 48, 1200–1207.

Schuetze, P., Eiden, R.D., & Danielewicz, S. (2009). 'The association between prenatal cocaine exposure and physiological regulation at 13 months of age'. *Journal of Child Psychology and Psychiatry*, 50, 1401–1409.

Shankman, S.A., Lewinsohn, P.M., Klein, D.N., Small, J.W., Seeley, J.R., & Altman, S.E. (2009). 'Subthreshold conditions as precursors for full syndrome disorders: A

15-year longitudinal study of multiple diagnostic classes'. *Journal of Child Psychology and Psychiatry*, 50, 1485–1494.
Sturgess, W., & Selwyn, J. (2007). 'Supporting the placements of children adopted out of care'. *Clinical Child Psychology and Psychiatry*, 12, 13–28.
Swanson, J.D., & Wadhwa, P.M. (2008). 'Developmental origins of child mental health disorders'. *Journal of Child Psychiatry and Psychology*, 10, 1009–1019.
Tarren-Sweeney, M. (2006). 'Patterns of aberrant eating among pre-adolescent children in foster care'. *Journal of Abnormal Child Psychology*, 34, 623–634.
——(2007). 'The Assessment Checklist for Children – ACC: A behavioural rating scale for children in foster, residential and kinship care'. *Children and Youth Services Review*, 30, 1–25.
——(2008). 'Predictors of problematic sexual behaviour among children with complex maltreatment histories'. *Child Maltreatment*, 13, 182–198.
Thapar, A., & Rutter, M. (2009). 'Do prenatal risk factors cause psychiatric disorder? Be wary of causal claims'. *British Journal of Psychiatry*, 195, 100–101.
van der Kolk, B. (2005). 'Developmental trauma disorder'. *Psychiatric Annals*, 35, 401–408.
van der Kolk, B., Roth, S., Pelcovitz, D., Sunday, S., & Spinazzola, J. (2005). 'Disorders of extreme stress: The empirical foundation of a complex adaptation to trauma'. *Journal of Traumatic Stress*, 18, 389–399.
Volkmar, F.R., State, M., & Klin, A. (2009). 'Autism and autistic spectrum disorders: Diagnostic issues for the coming decade'. *Journal of Child Psychology and Psychiatry*, 50, 108–115.
Woodcock Ross, J., Hooper, L., Stenhouse, E., & Sheaff, R. (2009). 'What are childcare social workers doing in relation to infant mental health? An exploration of professional ideologies and practice preferences within an inter-agency context'. *British Journal of Social Work*, 39, 1008–1025.
Zeanah, C.E. (1996). 'Beyond insecurity: A reconceptualization of attachment disorders of infancy'. *Journal of Consulting and Clinical Psychology*, 64, 42–52.
Zeanah, C., Sceerings, M., Boris, N., Heller, S., Smyke, A., & Trapani, J. (2004). 'Reactive Attachment Disorder in maltreated toddlers'. *Child Abuse & Neglect*, 28, 877–888.
Zeanah, C.E., & Smyke, A.T. (2008). 'Attachment disorders in relation to deprivation'. In M. Rutter et al. (eds) *Rutter's child and adolescent psychiatry* (5th ed.) (pp. 906–915). Oxford: Blackwell.
Zeanah, C.H., Smyke, A.T., & Settles, L. (2006). 'Children in orphanages'. In K. McCartney & D. Phillips (Eds.), *Blackwell handbook of early childhood development* (pp. 224–254). Malden, MA: Blackwell Publishing.
Zilberstein, K. (2006) 'Clarifying core characteristics of attachment disorders: A review of current research and theory'. *American Journal of Orthopsychiatry*, 76, 55–63.

11 The making and breaking of relationships

Organisational and clinical questions in establishing a family life for looked after children[1]

John Simmonds

Summary

The mental health of children in public care has received considerable attention in recent years. There are significant differences in the prevalence rates compared to children living at home and not in public care and these are added to by other adverse lifestyle issues. Considerable attention has been focused on the importance of stable and secure placements supported by access to a range of services including education, health and mental health. Identifying and classifying mental health needs proves to be challenging as the child's genetic inheritance, pre- and post-birth experiences, including maltreatment, interact with the uncertainty and delays commonly associated with child protection processes, action in the legal system and the difficulty in establishing secure and permanent placements. Clinical need is also related to the age of the child and the reasons they came into care and the length of time they remain. A case illustrating many of these issues, publicly reported in a court judgement, is used as the basis for exploring the complexity for the identified child in understanding and making sense of their experiences as placement plans are made for them.[2] These are used to explore the difficulties in establishing clinical protocols such as those recently published in the UK and USA. Particular emphasis is given to the issues faced by children and their carers in establishing new family relationships where they are combine the opportunities available from that family and the long shadow cast from previous family and 'in care' experiences especially where these are traumatic and conflicted in origin.

Introduction

For any child or young person to leave their family of origin to be cared for by public authorities, whether temporarily or permanently, is, for the majority, going to be a difficult and unwelcome experience. There are likely to be profound feelings of separation and loss, anxiety about what is happening and why, and fears for the future. These may be mitigated by relief at leaving a dangerous or unsatisfactory family home, but that relief will be moderated by the other feelings that are part of the mix. At the heart of this there are powerful issues about the breaking and making of relationships for the child and the consequences this may have for the child's development especially those many aspects of development that are determined by the sensory, relational world that shapes the interacting forces of the child, their family and the world of opportunity. In terms of mental health the issues couldn't be starker. In a wide ranging study of 1039 looked after children age 5 to 17 from local authorities in England, 466 were assessed as having a mental health disorder (Meltzer, Gatward, Corbin, Goodman, & Ford, 2003). By far, the greater numbers of these were assessed to have a clinically significant conduct disorder (37%), while a smaller number (12%) were identified as having an emotional disorder and a smaller number still, hyperkinetic disorders (7%). In comparison to an earlier survey (Meltzer, Gatward, with Goodman, & Ford, 2000) of 5–10-year-old children living with their parents or other parental figures and not the responsibility of the state, the rates for clinically significant disorders were 8% in private households compared to 42% in the looked after children cohort. For young people between the ages of 11 and 15 the rates were 49% compared to 11%. One significant finding in the looked after sample was the decrease in the rate of mental health disorders in those children and young people associated with their length of time in placement. For those children in their current placement for less than a year, the overall rate was 49% while for those in their current placement for 5 years or more it was 31%. Stability of placement, a central policy initiative in England, is a clear if complex indicator of positive outcomes, although what creates stability is an unanswered question from this study. Apart from clinically significant disorders, the study also identified other lifestyle issues that are generally identified to be detrimental to health. The rates of smoking in 11–15-year-olds were three times higher than those not looked after at 27% and if the young person had a mental disorder, then the rate was over 50%. Increased prevalence was also found in relation to alcohol consumption and drug use, particularly cannabis, and where there was a mental disorder 19% had used cannabis in the last month compared to 6% who did not have a mental disorder. Similar issues were raised in relation to young people's combined use of cigarettes, alcohol and illegal drugs. Heightened rates of sexual activity were also reported. These figures compare to a similar study in the USA (Burns et al., 2004) where, using the CBCL, in cases of children and young people age between 2 and 14 reported for maltreatment, 47.9% of the sample of 3803 were shown to have clinically significant emotional and behavioural problems.

These are disturbing figures and have been important in raising questions about the needs of looked after children and young people in respect of their mental and other health needs, both in terms of assessment and intervention. There are messages here for local authorities in the way that they assess, plan, make decisions and then arrange and deliver services. There are messages here for the health service in the way that they assess, intervene and organise their services, particularly mental health services. And there are messages for a range of other service providers – education, lawyers and the courts and foster carers and adopters. Each has a part to play, either in the prevention or treatment of mental health disorders in looked after children and young people. The difficulty is in identifying what part these services play and indeed what the concept of mental health or ill health means for the work that they do. There are a number of issues that should be taken into account. The Meltzer study quite properly based its questionnaire design on diagnostic research criteria as set out in ICD-10: 'clinically recognisable ... symptoms or behaviour associated with considerable distress and substantial interference with personal functioning' (Melzer et al., 2003, p. 9) However, the justification for using an established set of definitions is preceded in the report by a reference to the NHS Health Advisory Service's (1995) concern about the need, firstly, to reconcile the potential for stigmatising the child by the use of terms such as mental disorder while accurately describing clinical conditions in order to helpfully intervene. Secondly, there is a need to identify those conditions which reside in the child and those that act as external stressors on the child which need resolution in their own right, such as maltreating parents or the absence of a family life. In any assessment process in child and adolescent mental health, providing services that are non-stigmatizing and non-blaming while being specific, accurate and reliable, that support the child through their distress and troubles while addressing poor parenting or lack of planning are clearly important, although in practice this may be very difficult to do in a coherent way. With children separated from their birth parents and looked after by the state, this may be particularly challenging as the resolution of the issues concerning the child's future care runs alongside the immediate need to fully care for a child who will almost inevitably be in a distressed state brought on by the fact of separation from their birth parents and birth family and whatever immediate and past factors led to this. The resolution of these issues will be determined by the work of local authority children's services, the family courts and a range of other professionals and services. While it is usual to think of these parts of the system as playing a child centred role driven by values of justice, rights, equality, evidence and outcomes, the system in practice is often caught up in disputes, misunderstanding, resource constraints, defensiveness and delay. It is itself a complex relational world that plays itself out either under the influence of the families that it works with, or through its own patterns of rules, relationships and patterns of engagement. If families are caught up in their own histories and patterns of resistance, avoidance, disorganisation or trauma, so can state systems although it is rare for this to be openly acknowledged in quite the same way (Norgrove, 2011; Brandon, Sidebotham, et al, 2012). If the mental health of children and their families is one core issue, so might the mental health of the systems designed to help? This idea runs throughout the following discussion.

Modelling the care system by age and need

One of the most important issues in understanding the meaning of mental health and the objectives of services in promoting, preventing or addressing mental health needs for children in public care is recognising the complexity of what the care system is and what it is required to do. Given that the age span of children is from birth to 18 and for some, into early adulthood, defining the mental health component is complex. This is compounded by the fact that the age when a child enters the system, the length of time they remain, the pathway through the system including moves from carer to carer and their exit out of the system are all variables that impact on development and outcome. In a study of 13 English local authorities and 7399 children (Sinclair, Baker, Lee, & Gibbs, 2007), a model is proposed which explores stability based on the age at which the child first entered care. The model makes a distinction between those children who first enter care under the age of 11 (43%) and those between the ages of 11 and 18 (57%). In the adolescent age group a number of other sub-groups were identified – those who first entered care under 11 and continued to be cared for into adolescence (26%), those that first came into care as a result of abuse (9%), those that came into care because of a serious breakdown in their family of origin (14%), and lastly unaccompanied asylum-seeking children (5%). Another much smaller group was identified as those with complex and high-level needs (3%). Each group was different, especially in terms of the degree to which they achieved a permanent and stable placement. Age and need clearly influenced this. Young children either returned home, although some re-entered or left care through being adopted, or remained in care for a considerable period of time. For those children who returned home or were adopted, the care system is a transitional phase en route to a stable and secure family life. For those children under 11 who remain, the care system takes on the responsibility of parenting them, usually in foster care. Many of these children then continue to be parented by the care system as they make a transition into and progress through their adolescent years. The study looked at child outcomes in terms of both long-term stability and well-being, with well-being a factor that was strongly related to a child's age, their age at entry to care, the experience of being returned home and then returned to care and then, the quality of the placement that they were in. Where children were under 11, their placements were as likely to last irrespective of the quality of the placement. This then identified a number of children in stable placements but where their underlying distress was acute. For those children entering care over 11 because of abuse or family breakdown, their needs were marked by high levels of challenging behaviour and difficulties at school. These young people were not in a position to return home, or because of their challenging behaviour, there were significant difficulties in establishing them in secure, stable placements. The placements they were in were identified as being poorly equipped to positively address their difficulties. Forty-nine per cent of abused adolescents had placements that had lasted for less than six months and 60% of adolescent entrants. Unaccompanied asylum-seeking young people posed a different set of issues because of the overriding question of their immigration status. Their claim for asylum marks out their need for refuge from political persecution or oppression and in that sense, a 'positive choice' to enter the UK and the care system. But the multiple traumas they may have experienced prior to departure, during their journey and on arrival will produce their own set of complex mental health issues that do bear direct comparison to UK children. Even so, 40% had had placements that had lasted less than six months.

Designing a mental health system for children in public care faces a complex task in identifying its contribution to the multiple responsibilities that each of these groups in this study creates. As Meltzer identifies, clinical need will run throughout this group in many different ways (Melzer et al., 2003). The responsibility to establish a loving family that will endure throughout childhood and beyond for a 6-month-old is quite different to meeting the needs of an unaccompanied asylum seeker with Post-traumatic Stress Disorder facing deportation. The mental health issues for the 6-month- old should not be underestimated with heightened risk from genetic factors, prenatal exposure to legal and illegal substances, alcohol and nicotine and probably six months of high levels of stress brought about by the systemically generated factors of the legal, children's and health services. But is the arrangement of an alternative family placement for a child, a mental health intervention? Clearly it is and of a radical kind but it is not usually primarily defined as such as it is the responsibility of children's services whose primary conceptual set is defined by the Assessment of Children in Need Framework (Department of Health, 2000). Mental health need will primarily be defined as the need for a loving family and met through the complex processes that enable that. The part that dedicated mental health services will play in that assessment and family finding process is likely to be limited and may be absent in making a proactive contribution although public health guidance issued by the National Institute for Health and Clinical Excellence (2010) develops this issue quite significantly. It may be that issues such as a child's attachment security or the adopter's attachment classification have been assessed as a part of their approval. And for older children, it may also be that a child's need for therapeutic intervention has been assessed and arranged. But the issue of the creation of a family around the child, temporarily or permanently, as the primary therapeutic intervention linking children's services including education and CAMHS is not well articulated. This is so despite the statutory requirement in the Adoption and Children

Act 2002 in England and Wales, there should be an assessment of support needs including therapeutic needs. It is by no means the case that therapeutic interventions have not been developed or are unavailable and there have been English pilots of evidenced-based interventions imported from the Blueprints Project such as Functional Family Therapy (Alexander et al., 1998), the Nurse-Family Partnership (Olds, Hill, Mihalic, & O'Brien, 1998) and Multi-Dimensional Treatment Foster Care (Price et al., 2008). There are also national roll-outs of evidence-based interventions such as Fostering Changes (Bachmann, 2011), KEEP (Price, 2008) and evidence from RCTs such as Enhancing Adoptive Parenting (Rushton & Monck, 2009; Rushton & Upright, 2012).

An (imagined) case example

Some of these issues are exemplified by a case heard in the Court of Appeal in 2007 (R (Children) [2007] EWCA Civ 139). There is nothing particularly unusual in the case itself although its complexity and the issues at stake in relation to the long-term welfare and placement of three children will be very familiar to most people with experience of making plans and decisions for children coming into local authority care. The issue of child development and mental health run throughout the case but the way in which a mental health perspective influences how decisions were taken and plans made to meet the developmental and health needs of the children concerned is difficult to identify.

The case concerned a grandmother's application for a Special Guardianship Order against the local authority's plan to place the three children for adoption. The three children were Joey, a boy aged 8; Cheryl, a girl aged 5; and Robert, a boy aged 3. The three children had the same mother – Caroline. Joey's father was Sam although he believed him to be Ashley, the father of the two younger children. Ashley also had children through another relationship which continued while he was married to Caroline. The membership of this family and their relationships was, as is often the case with children who become looked after, complex (see Figure 11.1). Ashley and Caroline's relationship was violent and chaotic and on one occasion Caroline needed to live in a refuge. Joey was seriously affected by this. He was caught up and injured in some of the incidents and observed others where his mother was attacked. Alcohol and amphetamine use by the parents played a part in stoking the fires of a tempestuous family life. Not surprisingly, Joey's school attendance was erratic. Eventually, the children were made subject to a Police Protection Order following the arrest of Ashley after a fire was started outside the family home and Caroline was arrested for being drunk and disorderly. Initially, the local authority placed the children in different foster care placements and then eventually together. The local authority's plan was either to place the children for adoption or to place them with the maternal grandmother, Jean. Jean was somebody who had

200 John Simmonds

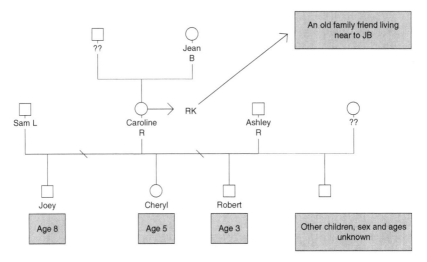

Figure 11.1 Joey's family tree

been assessed as having many 'positives' including her commitment to the children and the children's love of her. At the same time she had had a very difficult life having been in care herself and involved in a number of violent relationships and there was concern about her capacity to overcome these difficulties and provide a stable home life for her grandchildren.

There were a number of concerns when the court of first instance considered the case:

- Joey was seen to need therapy to enable him to move on which would take 6–8 months.
- Finding an adoption placement for him was likely to prove difficult.
- There was no plan to inform Joey of the identity of his real father Sam.
- There was no assessment of the sibling relationships.
- There was no assessment of each of the child's needs.
- There was no plan to tell the children of their other half siblings.

As a result, the case was adjourned to give time to address these issues and in particular for a full assessment of the maternal grandmother Jean's capacity to provide a stable family life for the children including the question of her safely managing contact between the children and their parents. There was also a very real practical problem in that she lived in a one-bedroom flat in a different part of the country and her local authority were not prepared to do anything to address the housing problem.

A positive report from a consultant clinical psychologist convinced the local authority that the plan should be for the maternal grandmother to become the carer for the three children. As a result, Jean was to have increased contact with the three children, to look after them during the summer holidays and then they were to move in with her and start school in the new term. However, there was continuing anxiety about Jean's relationship with her daughter Caroline and especially her capacity to appropriately protect Joey from his mother. Joey was very anxious about being exposed to his mother's behaviour and the threat that she posed to him, as well as his (step) father, Ashley. It was therefore decided not to inform the children of the plan for them to live with Jean and to continue to restrict the contact between the children and their mother. The difficulties of doing this were noted in the judgement when Joey met DB, a friend of his maternal grandmother in his grandmother's home and was very upset by what he said to him. In fact Joey's continuing worries about his mother and partner and his expressed wish not to live with his mother although to retain contact with her caused the planned move to be postponed. However, the local authority social workers were very encouraged when the children returned from a two-week visit to Jean which had gone very well. Joey was also seen to be very upset on leaving his grandmother to return to the foster carers. Following a positive visit to the children by Jean at the foster carer's home, the social worker expressed the view that they had 'cracked it' and the placement with Jean was likely 'to be successful'.

Sadly, this proved not to be the case. At the foster home, Cheryl falsely accused Joey of hitting her. The foster father supported Cheryl although he knew her accusation to be false. He had decided that Joey needed to be 'taught a lesson about the perils of lying' and wanted him to experience what it felt like to be 'punished unfairly'. Joey responded with great upset to the foster father's chastisement of him 'grabbing his head in his own hands and disclosing that his mother Caroline had been present at his grandmothers during their two-week holiday', something that was expressly forbidden. During a visit by the social worker, Joey confirmed his report that his mother was present at his grandmother's and reiterated that he did not want to go to live with his grandmother. Subsequently he refused to see her and tore up a letter, cards and destroyed a birthday present from her. However, Joey's accusation that his mother was present during his two-week stay with Jean turned out not to be true. But his continuing distress as well as the uncertainty caused by the accusation, resulted in the local authority changing their plan and deciding that the children should be placed for adoption.

The Court of Appeal upheld the local authority's plan that the children should be placed for adoption but it is clear that this is not the end of the story. The difficulties of putting the plan for the three children into action are abundantly clear. Salvaging anything positive for the three children out of lifetime of maltreatment, uncertainty and disruption is extraordinary challenging. The case illustrates the importance of taking a mental health perspective in doing this but it also illustrates a number of problems in identifying what the nature of mental health means in these kinds of narratives for both professionals and family members. Some of these are to do with the problem of establishing what has actually happened over a child's lifetime. Facts are critical in most professional contexts and core to understanding the nature of the problem and identifying solutions. At the same time most professionals in these kinds of situations rely heavily on a range of soft information. As this case illustrates, soft information is complex not just because it is difficult to assign validity and significance to it but because it is constructed and manipulated depending on the circumstances and intentions of the parties involved. For professionals, who to believe, what is the truth, who is safe and who is dangerous, what is the best thing to do now and how to predict let alone control what happens in the future including managing the interaction of the complex variables is challenging. Becoming involved as a professional can feel like being sucked into a nightmare of distortions and misunderstandings where the ground threatens to fall away at every turn. Retaining any sense of objectivity, rigour or indeed hope in the face of such complexity is extremely difficult. This case example illustrates this very clearly.

But if this is so for professionals where there is an expectation of a dispassionate child-centred stance and recourse to expertise, training and support, what about the perspective of children in such circumstances. What might it be like if we tried to imagine this story from Joey's perspective? And imagination may be all that we have to link the various components of the story together. For Joey, the people who are meant to love you and keep you safe, your mother and father are not safe as they subject you and each other to violence, conflict and other unimaginably terrifying ordeals from the moment you are born. You come to see your mother on the one hand as a victim of your father but on the other she is also a perpetrator, with her alcohol- and drug-driven out-of-control behaviour which is frightening to watch and terrifying to be on the receiving end of. In fact your father is not your father and the adults who are supposed to have the emotional resources and maturity to tell you this painful news, can't. This nightmare of wanting to be loved and trying to love back but being confronted by hate lasts for five long years, the only years you have known. And then after a particularly frightening incident, the police come and take you away – what have you done wrong? Are they going to put you in prison? But no, they put you by yourself with people you have never met and just as you are getting to know them and possibly like them, you are taken away again and go to live with some more people but this time you are reunited with your (half) brother and sister, a fact nobody has had the courage to tell you about either. But is this placement a temporary arrangement or will you go back to your mother and (step)father? Should you feel any loyalty to your mum and dad as you get to like these new people who feed you, make sure you are properly clothed and regularly take you to school on time with everything you need? But if you like these people too much will your mum and dad think you are being disloyal and about to betray them? 'Do you' or 'can you' or 'should you' love these new adults – have they finally rescued you from the nightmare of your parents or will you find yourself becoming a victim to these people's yet to be revealed erratic and terrifying behaviour?

It has been suggested to you that 'focussed therapy' will sort all these dilemmas and questions out and you will then be able to settle in your mind and get on with life. But the plan is to see if things can be worked out with grandma whom you like and maybe love but what about her loyalty to her own daughter, your mother and your mother's friend? Is grandma to be trusted? Will or can she rescue you or is she trapping you into believing that she is a rescuer from the nightmare when really she will again make you again into a victim of your mother's erratic and violent behaviour? And then you learn that your social workers believe that they have 'cracked it' because you liked staying with your grandmother over the summer and her visiting you. The social workers think they have detected that you do love your grandma. However, they have not told you that they believe that 'they have cracked it' although you know that they think this even though they haven't told you.

Then your sister accuses you of hitting her although you didn't and your rescuer foster father thinks that in order to teach you a lesson about the importance of telling the truth, it is better to tell a lie. You break down in despair as these people who are supposed to be sane adults are driving you mad and you clasp your head in your hands in sheer disbelief at the manner in which they express their adult sanity.

Taking a child's perspective on experiences like this is a very difficult thing to do. A lot is being asked of them to resolve dilemmas and conflicts that adults find it difficult to get their heads around. There is nothing in his case that lends itself to easy resolution and at the point at which the judgement was reported, there was some way to go. There can be no doubt that Joey and his brother and sister need to be in a stable and loving home where the adults understand that he is conflicted, distrustful, frightened and has had a very bad start in life. He will undoubtedly continue to show these conflicts, his distrust, his fear and the impact of his bad start in life for many years to come. It can be said that Joey knows what it means to:

- love and like your grandmother but not want to live with her.
- feel a sense of loyalty to your mother and never want to see her again.
- want a settled life but feel chaos inside.
- want to forget the past but remember it all the time.

Any professional reading about an 8-year-old like this will be drawn to thinking about a range of mental health issues arising from his genetic inheritance, his early life experiences and his time in care. In planning and deciding a placement, Joey's needs and those of his half siblings must be clearly understood and this must include having access to a well-functioning set of child development services. Core to this is an understanding of the nature of Joey's mental health needs and the kind of service provision that might address this.

A systemic approach to assessing and intervening in the mental health of looked after children

A conference in 2007 in the USA, Best Practices for Mental Health in Child Welfare, identified a number of issues in need of a solution: the gap between need and the provision of services, poor identification of mental health needs, the importance of evidence-based interventions and the overuse of psychotropic medication. The conference proposed a series of linked conceptual and organisational issues together with a set of guidelines as a solution to the problems identified above (Romanelli et al., 2009). These included:

Screening and assessment

1. Initial screening for emergent risk within 72 hours of entry to care.
2. Screening for on-going mental health service needs within 30 days of admission.
3. A comprehensive mental health assessment within 60 days for those receiving a positive screening using evidence-based instruments administered by qualified mental health practitioners.
4. Regular informal screening by the child's caseworker for mental health needs.

Interventions

1. Must be evidence-based or 'promising interventions' with adherence to evidence-based practice.
2. Should be individualised and strengths-based and reflect the child's permanency plan and include the child's current and past carers.
3. Should be delivered in partnership between child welfare and mental health providers.
4. Should track outcomes including psycho-social functioning, placement stability, permanency and client satisfaction.

A further set of nine guidelines concern psychopharmacologic treatments.

There is a strong argument for the development of protocols such as this and similar guidance developed by the National Institute for Clinical Excellence in the U.K. (National Institute for Health and Clinical Excellence, 2010). The early screening for mental health difficulties and comprehensive assessment of those difficulties at the point of entry to care seemed to be missing in Joey's case. Understanding these in the short term and long term will be critical to meeting his needs. However, there are also real difficulties in knowing exactly what early screening might focus on in his case. He has been separated from his mother, his (step)father and two half siblings by the police. He has immediate experience of fire setting outside his home allegedly, by his (step)father and the arrest of his mother. As immediately disturbing as any of this is likely to be for him, it is also clear that this is only one more episode in a lifetime of adversity. It is likely that his physical health, educational development, capacity for friendship and opportunities to engage in a range of age appropriate activities will have suffered. At the same time, some children develop remarkable resilience in the face of such adversity. But even if this is so, a predicted and expected response to these circumstances will be one of immense distress, confusion and anxiety tempered by some relief at being removed from the source of stress. But how this is manifested in behaviour may be something that is much more difficult to predict given Joey's need to have established strategies to survive past traumas. Assessing Joey in this crisis might be important but that may be different to assessing him as the immediate crisis abates and the longer-term issues come to the fore. The immediate impact and responsibility for addressing this will be with children's services and the social workers responsible for Joey. This will also include designated looked after children paediatricians and nurse specialists responsible for undertaking initial health assessments. Although these assessments should be 'Joey focussed', the responsibility to collect medical evidence that might be required for legal proceedings – both in the criminal or civil courts will have their own momentum. The range and number of professionals involved at this early and later stage is likely to be high (Conway, 2009) and considerable effort and expenditure is likely to be tied up in this. However, the primary responsibility for meeting Joey's needs will be with the foster carer. They will be above all, the immediate primary therapeutic agent and their capacity to form a relationship with him and create the conditions that can address Joey's needs are paramount. But as is so often the case, those likely to be the most influential through their capacity to relate to Joey are also likely to be the most marginalised in terms of status, support, training and reward.

In the longer term, Joey's primary needs including his mental health status are related to and will be determined by the question of 'With whom should he live?' and 'Who should parent him?' The legal proceedings are primarily concerned with this question and establishing the 'best' answer to this difficult question. Whatever and whoever this is, the task these parental figures will face will be strongly determined by the state of Joey's development, including his capacity to make relationships in the context of a new found family intimacy and the influence of his past experiences and expectations on these new opportunities. Parenting him well will involve both addressing the complexities of developmental catch-up where this is possible and adaptation of the carers to his emotional and behavioural survival strategies. There are also a set of 'secondary' questions about the continuation and influence of his birth family relationships – with his mother, stepfather and father, his half siblings – both those that he has come to experience as full siblings and those that he does not yet know of at all. His relationship with his interim foster family is also significant given that he has spent just under 40% of his life with them. Joey's development and his mental health are intimately connected with the nature and quality of the relationships he has with all of these people. The incident with the foster carer demonstrates just how challenging this can be. At one level this incident might be considered to be a routine episode in the challenge of parenting – a squabble between siblings and the frustration of a father figure trying to exercise some control over a child's lying – but in this instance it becomes a life course changing turning point. It is the straw that breaks the camel's back and brings to the fore the distress of a child who cannot make sense of the unpredictability and distortions of the adult world. His survival strategies, whether they are lying, destroying presents or tearing up cards, are his strategies and they are presumably well embedded in his neurological make-up (De Bellis, 2005) and his personality. These issues are clearly inside Joey as an individual and a comprehensive mental health assessment undertaken at the appropriate time of the type recommended in the protocol may come up with a formulation of this. But the rebuke of his foster father clearly indicates that many of the issues Joey faces as an individual are reactions to, interpretations of and responses from his relational world. The incident attains its meanings when it is considered in the immediate context of the foster father and Joey's (half) sister Cheryl but they are a part of a wider emotionally charged relational world made up of his grandmother, mother and other family members. Beyond that there is also a similar emotionally charged relational world made up of social workers, psychologists, lawyers and other professionals although it is not usual to describe it in this way. In each of these relational worlds people are trying to make sense of their experience from a personal and/or professional perspective. The primary influences on this I suggest are thoughts, feelings and responsibilities for the breaking and making of relationships where the experience of relating is full of risk. 'Who is safe?', 'Who cares?', 'Does this feel good or reassuring?', 'Does anybody know how bad I feel?', 'Who knows what this feels like for me?' Feelings of guilt, shame and anger and hope, comfort and understanding are overarching themes in the pursuit of a family life for Joey as well as the day-to-day questions that structure his experience of relating. Every individual who makes up the system responsible for answering the challenging questions of how to break and make relationships for Joey will be faced by troubling feelings stirred up by this profound responsibility to get it 'right' with the real fear of getting it wrong. Guilt, shame and anger are as much a part of the professional world when the consequences of the decisions that are made in the process of breaking and making relationships impact on children in ways that are lifelong. That responsibility may become unbearable especially when it results in having to bear the consequences of thinking, feeling and doing things in life-changing ways similar to that of the foster father.

    The development and publication of guidance in both the USA and the UK in relation to services for looked after children are important. The NIHCE Public Health Guidance stresses the importance of 'organisations, professionals and carers work together to deliver high quality care, stable placements and nurturing relationships for looked-after children and young people' (page 5). This is further articulated in a set of principles and values which are undoubtedly child centred and more specifically 52 recommendations to support their implementation. Throughout, there is a realistic emphasis on evidence-based practice, a strong drive towards inter-agency working and the development of effective commissioning to improve standards. It is a rational presentation of a complex, long-term organisational change and improvement programme. There are numerous professionals in CAMH and in children's services and the courts dedicated to this with many examples of creative, thoughtful and effective services. However, it is also important to recognise that the weight of establishing and delivering an effective response to the issues presented by children like Joey falls heavily on the 'ordinariness' of family life and what adopters and foster carers can do to remedy the poor starts in life that many children have experienced. The support of CAMHS and the contribution of a mental health and developmental perspective for them is critical. But observing the working of the system as a whole suggests, as Joey's case illustrates, that creating a relational therapeutic community around the child is an extraordinary difficult thing to do. A system that is primarily concerned with the fundamental breaking and making of primary relationships can itself be infected by doubt, shame, anxiety and guilt and can act in ways that actually create traumatic conditions on top of those the child has already experienced in their family. The linkages between people and professionals that should create meaningful and thoughtful communication about children and their circumstances can be used to attribute blame or punish, as the incident with the foster carer demonstrates. Linkages between professionals that should facilitate unbearable feelings of loss, betrayal and guilt being put into words can as easily break down, as they have in Joey's family. The various protocols, standards and guidance barely touch on the relational dynamics of the breaking and making of family relationships. The prescription of a standardised consumer-driven service delivery framework is a start but seems significantly at odds with the issues presented in this case. Effective mental health interventions for birth or alternative families struggling with overwhelming odds need to take into account the relational and emotional issues that drive them. Whether protocols such as Best Practices or the NIHCE guidance where the use of standardised instruments to identify clinical need in order to deliver standardised, evidence-based intervention packages are sufficient needs to be debated. But if and as that happens, Joey and his siblings can't wait.

Notes

1 A version of this chapter was previously published as: Simmonds, J. (2010). The making and breaking of relationships: Organizational and clinical questions in providing services for looked after children? *Clinical Child Psychology and Psychiatry*, 15(4), 601–612.

2 These names are made up for ease of discussion. The judges in the case made it clear that nothing should be published that identifies the children or others in the case and this has been strictly adhered to in the facts reported here. Those facts discussed are on public record.

References

Alexander, J., Barton, C., et al. (1998). *Functional family therapy: Blueprints for violence prevention, book three*. Boulder, CO: Center for the Study and Prevention of Violence, Institute of Behavioral Science, University of Colorado.

Bachmann, K., K. Blackeby, et al. (2011). *Fostering changes: How to improve relationships and manage difficult behaviour*. London, BAAF

Brandon, M., P. Sidebotham, et al. (2012). *New learning from serious case reviews*. Dept. of Education, University of East Anglia and University of Warwick.

Burns, B., Phillips, S., et al. (2004). 'Mental health need and access to mental health services by youths involved with child welfare: A national survey'. *Journal of the American Academy of Child and Adolescent Psychiatry*, 43(8), 960–970.

Conway, P. (2009). 'Falling between minds: The effects of unbearable experiences on multi-agency communication in the care system'. *Adoption and Fostering*, 33, 18–29.

De Bellis, M. (2005). 'The psychobiology of neglect'. *Child Maltreatment*, 10(2), 150–172.

Department of Children, Schools and Families & Department of Health (2008). *Children and young people in mind: The final report of the National CAMHS Review*. London: Department of Health. Available at: http://www.dcsf.gov.uk/CAMHSreview/downloads/CAMHSReview-Bookmark.pdf (accessed 16 February 2010).

——(2004). *National service framework for children, young people and maternity services: The mental health and psychological well-being of children and young people*. London: Department of Health.

Department of Health (2000). *Framework for the assessment of children in need and their families*. London: HMSO.

Loxterkamp, L. (2009). 'Contact and truth: The unfolding predicament in adoption and fostering'. *Clinical Child Psychology and Psychiatry*, 14(3), 423–435.

Meltzer, H., Gatward, R., et al. (2003). *The mental health of young people looked after by local authorities in England*. London: HMSO.

Meltzer, H., Gatward, R., with Goodman, R., & Ford, T. (2000). *The mental health of children and adolescents in Great Britain: Summary report*. London: HMSO.

National Institute for Health and Clinical Excellence (2010) *Promoting the quality of life of looked-after children and young people*: Public Health Guidance 28, NIHCE and SCIE.

NHS Health Advisory Service (1995) *Child and adolescent mental health services: Together we stand. The commissioning, role and management of child and adolescent mental health services*. London: HMSO.

Norgrove, D. (2011). *Family Justice Review: Final Report*. Ministry of Justice, Crown Copyright.

Olds, D., Hill, P., Mihalic, S., & O'Brien, R. (1998). *Nurse-family partnership: Blueprints for violence prevention, book seven*. Boulder, CO: Centre for the Study and Prevention of Violence, Institute of Behavioural Science, University of Colorado.

Pallett, P., Blackeby, K., Yule, W., Weissman, R., & Scott, S. (2005). *Fostering changes: How to improve relationships and manage difficult behaviour*. London: BAAF.

Price, J., Chamberlain, P., Landsverk, J., Reid, J., Leve, L., & Laurent, H. (2008). 'Effects of a foster parent training intervention on placement changes of children in foster care'. *Child Maltreatment*, 13(1), 64–75.

R *(Children) [2007] EWCA Civ 139*. Available from BAILII at: http://www.bailii.org/ew/cases/EWCA/Civ/2007/139.html (accessed 17 February 2010).

Romanelli, L., Landsverk, J., et al. (2009). 'Best practices for mental health in child welfare: Screening, assessment and treatment guidelines'. *Child Welfare*, SS(1), 163–188.

Ross, J. W., Hooper, L., Stenhouse, E., & Sheaff, R. (2009). 'What are child-care social workers doing in relation to infant mental health? An exploration of professional ideologies and practice preferences within an inter-agency context'. *British Journal of Social Work*, 39(6), 1008–1025.

Rushton, A., & Monck, E. (2009). *Enhancing adoptive parenting: A test of effectiveness*. London: BAAF.

Rushton, A., & H. Upright (2012). *Enhancing adoptive parenting: A parenting programme for use with new adopters of challenging children*. London: BAAF.

Sinclair, I., Baker, C., Lee, J., & Gibbs, I. (2007). *The pursuit of permanence: A study of the English care system*. London: Jessica Kingsley.

12 Principles for the design of mental health services for children and young people in care, and those adopted from care[1]

Michael Tarren-Sweeney

Summary

Much of what is written in this book points to the need for a clinical workforce that has much greater knowledge and skills for working with children with a history of alternate care, including those who are subsequently adopted. Standard child clinical conceptualisation, assessment methods and formulations miss the mark for these vulnerable populations in a number of critical ways. This final chapter proposes ten principles to guide the design of mental health services for children in care, and those adopted from care. Effective specialisation in child welfare work by clinical child psychologists, psychotherapists and psychiatrists, requires: (i) specialised knowledge and skills; (ii) a shift from traditional clinical practice to a *clinical/psychosocial-developmental* scope of practice; and (iii) a strong advocacy role. To support such specialised practice, service design should be guided by: (iv) a primary – specialist care nexus, that includes universal, comprehensive assessments; (v) a shift from acute care to preventative, long-term engagement and monitoring; (vi) integration within the social care milieu; (vii) a shift from exclusion to active ownership of these client groups; (viii) normalisation strategies; and (ix) alignment of services for these client groups. Finally, it is argued that mental health service provision for these vulnerable groups is strengthened by policy that promotes (x) 'whole of government' accountability for their mental health needs.

Why should we re-think mental health services for children in (and adopted from) care?

The present chapter's focus is limited to western jurisdictions in which foster and kinship care are the predominant forms of care. While specialised mental health services for child welfare populations have been established in some countries, no western jurisdiction has yet developed an integrated model of clinical practice that adequately addresses the parameters set out by various authors in this book. What has been realised to date has been largely piecemeal, initiated in the main by a small number of visionary clinicians. There are positive signs of some governments working in the right direction, as seen for example with England's 'Every Child Matters' programme (Great Britain: Department for Children Schools and Families and Department of Health, 2009), and the development of inter-government health and education services for children in care in New South Wales as part of the 'Keep Them Safe' initiative (New South Wales Government, 2010). Notwithstanding such progress, it can be argued that governments have generally underestimated the extent of change required, as evidenced by attempts to make existing service systems and professional practice models fit the needs of children in care. A recent review of CAMHS services in England (Great Britain: Department for Children Schools and Families and Department of Health, 2008) proposed a need for targeted mental health services for 'looked-after children', without considering whether such services are ideally developed within a CAMHS system. It contained no discussion on whether such services might be better placed elsewhere within the National Health Service (NHS), or outside of the NHS altogether (such as within the Department for Children, Schools and Families), except in relation to the commissioning of services by Children's Trusts.

The most visible shortcoming in the provision of mental health services for children in care, as well as those adopted from care (Sturgess & Selwyn, 2007), is insufficient capacity. This is despite these populations having high rates of service use relative to other disadvantaged children (Bellamy, Traube, & Gopalan, 2010; Sturgess & Selwyn, 2007). The prevalence of clinically significant mental health difficulties among these children is sufficiently high to warrant systematic assessment of their mental health service needs. In Chapter 11, John Simmonds outlines a population-based screening and assessment protocol designed by a committee of delegates at a U.S. 'Best Practices for Mental Health in Child Welfare' conference (Romanelli et al., 2009). These guidelines seem reasonable and well considered. Yet, it is unlikely that any state or country could sustain a 'whole of population' approach to detection and management of mental health difficulties among children in care without a large expansion of service capacity, regardless of whether the work is done by specialist alternate care teams, or generic child mental health services. It is known for example, that US children in care presently receive a disproportionate share of Medicaid public mental health services, relative to other disadvantaged child populations with high prevalence of mental health difficulties (Leslie et al., 2005), including maltreated children who remain in parental care.

Beyond questions of scale and capacity, it is apparent that publically funded, 'acute care' child and adolescent mental health services are poorly matched to the service needs of a disadvantaged child population presenting with complex attachment- and trauma-related psychopathology, and unstable living arrangements. Such children require greater continuity and certainty of care than acute care services are designed to provide. This requirement seems particularly ill-matched to acute care services that function within a 'managed care' environment (Leslie, Kelleher, Burns, Landsverk, & Rolls, 2003), or which are required to achieve high client turnover.

Thirdly, as outlined in Chapter 10 by Margaret DeJong, there are big question marks for this population around the coherence and validity of clinical formulations based on standard conceptualisations of psychopathology, and using standard assessment data. In 1996, I reviewed 110 clinical assessment reports sourced from 50 psychological records of children in care, and other child welfare clients, as part of the development of a mental health checklist for children in care and related populations. Most of these reports were written by psychologists and psychiatrists working in specialist public health services, child welfare and alternate care agencies, and private practice. The reports revealed considerable diagnostic disagreement and uncertainty, as well as a tendency to frame complex psychopathology as a series of discrete, co-morbid disorders. From a practice perspective, the accumulation of multiple and conflicting diagnoses provides little clarity or guidance for children's social workers, teachers and carers (DeJong, 2010). Whereas a little more than half of children in care have clinically significant mental health difficulties, cluster analyses of symptoms measured in the NSW Children in Care study identified 20% of children with complex attachment- and trauma-related psychopathology that is not adequately conceptualised within standard classification (Tarren-Sweeney, In Press).

Finally, amongst colleagues who provide clinical services for children in care and/or those adopted from care, there is reasonable consensus that standard psychological and pharmacological interventions appear less effective for these children. Yet, there are almost no research data describing the effectiveness of standard treatments for these children, while the effectiveness of interventions designed specifically for adopted or in care populations remains somewhat uncertain (see Chapter 3 for detailed coverage of this topic). In Chapter 2, Jennifer Bellamy and colleagues report their findings of an analysis of the effects of standard out-patient mental health treatment for a national sample of 439 children in long-term foster care, drawn from the US National Survey of Child and Adolescent Well-being (NSCAW). Their analysis controlled for a number of known or likely confounders, while change was measured from baseline and 18-month follow-up caregiver-reported Child Behaviour Checklist (CBCL) scores. They found that outpatient treatment had no independent effect on changes to CBCL scores, suggesting that collectively, interventions that constitute standard outpatient treatment in the US may not be effective (at least over this timeframe). A useful next step in this area of research is to examine the effectiveness of specific types of intervention for children in care, as provided through generic outpatient services. The evidence supporting various 'evidence-based' child psychological interventions is mostly limited to findings from clinical trials, in which treatment response has not been stratified by special population status. These findings may thus not generalise to children in care, and children adopted from care. For example, the mechanisms accounting for the characteristic inattention/over-activity of severely deprived children (Kreppner et al., 2001) may differ from those that account for other inattention/over-activity, in which case alternative treatments may be warranted. Generic treatment modalities are also mostly designed for discrete disorders rather than complex bio-psycho-social phenomena. Children in care are more likely to present with complex disorders (Tarren-Sweeney, 2008) that are less likely to respond to psychological treatments developed for discrete disorders, such as depression (National Institute for Clinical Excellence NICE, 2005).

Along similar lines, there has been little discussion about the potential for psychotherapy to harm children and young people in care. Fonagy and Bateman (2006) have speculated that traditional psychotherapies are harmful for some adults with Borderline Personality Disorder, due to iatrogenic mechanisms involving impaired mentalisation capacity, and the activation of their attachment systems within a therapeutic alliance. If there is substance to this, then it seems plausible that the sizeable proportion of children in care who have complex attachment- and trauma-related difficulties could be similarly vulnerable to experiencing harmful effects from a number of common psychotherapies. These considerations highlight a need for research on mental health treatment for children in care, and those adopted from care, and a parallel need for better informed treatment planning for these children.

Ten principles to guide the design of mental health services for children in care (and those adopted from care)

The following principles are meant to complement and extend on the body of ideas contained within existing clinical practice guidelines (Romanelli et al., 2009; Royal Australian & New Zealand College of Psychiatrists, 2008) and various government initiatives. They are also written as a partial response to the challenges raised in this book by John Simmonds, Kim Golding, and Margaret DeJong, leaving aside the design of psychosocial interventions for these special populations. The principles are arranged at three levels (summarised in Table 12.1): Level 1 – *Specialised practice*; Level 2 – *Service models*; and Level 3 – *Civil society*. These levels can be thought of as concentric spheres of influence on the lives of those children who receive services, the most proximal referring to clinicians and the parameters of specialised practice.

Level 1 – Specialised practice

Much of what is written in this book points to the need for a clinical workforce that has a deeper knowledge and skill set for working with children with a history of alternate care or other child welfare involvement. Existing child clinical training – whether it is through clinical psychology, child

214 Michael Tarren-Sweeney

Table 12.1 Summary of principles for guiding the design of mental health services for children in care (and those adopted from care)

Level 1: Specialised practice	
	(i) Specialised knowledge and skills
	(ii) Clinical/psychosocial-developmental scope of practice
	(iii) Advocacy
Level 2: Service models	
	(iv) Primary – specialist care nexus, and universal assessment
	(v) Preventative, long-term engagement and monitoring
	(vi) Integral part of social care milieu
	(vii) Active ownership
	(viii) Normalisation strategies
	(ix) Service alignment
Level 3: Civil society	
	(x) Whole of government accountability

psychotherapy, or child and adolescent psychiatry training schemes – does not adequately prepare trainees for understanding or working with these children. I propose that effective specialisation in child welfare work by psychologists, psychotherapists and psychiatrists, requires: specialised knowledge and skills; a shift from traditional clinical practice to what might be termed *clinical/psychosocial-developmental* scope of practice; and a strong advocacy role.

Specialised knowledge and skills

As outlined earlier in this chapter, standard child clinical conceptualisation, assessment methods and formulations miss the mark for these vulnerable populations in a number of critical ways. This is partly indicative of gaps in knowledge that have yet to be clarified through research. However, a lot has also been learned that is yet to be translated into standard clinical practice, including knowledge and skills that can increase clinicians' understanding of these children, and yield more accurate clinical formulations. In the main these have quite a specialised focus, requiring fairly detailed or intensive training. For this reason, it is more realistic to set our sights on developing specialised clinical workforces for child welfare work, than expanding the scope of standard clinical training. The development of specialised workforces requires both high-quality training, and the maintenance of specialist practice standards through professional bodies.

What then should be the main characteristics of specialised clinical practice with these populations? First, it should be guided by appropriate conceptual frameworks for formulating complex attachment- and trauma-related disorders, and the bio-psycho-social mechanisms and developmental pathways that determine the mental health of children with a history of care and/or maltreatment. The significance of early social adversity and attachment conditions on these populations' neurological and psychological development, points to complex, time-sensitive aetiological mechanisms. For these children more than others, it is essential that we incorporate new knowledge from developmental psychopathology research, and an ecological – transactional framework (e.g. Cicchetti et al. (2000)) into clinical reasoning and case hypothesis generation.

In addition to ecological enquiry, specialised clinical practice requires an improved conceptualisation of complex attachment- and trauma-related symptomatology manifested by these children (DeJong, 2010). While some work has been devoted to re-conceptualising such difficulties (Crittenden, 1997; O'Connor & Zeanah, 2003; van der Kolk, 2005) it may be several decades before we attain an empirically validated classification of attachment- and trauma-related mental health difficulties that accommodates a high degree of symptom complexity. Until that eventuates, I believe that specialised clinical practice requires both an understanding of the particular limitations of present diagnostic classifications in relation to these forms of psychopathology, and some modification of clinical reasoning and formulation to work around these limitations. One 'work-around' is employing a *profile approach* to the formulation of complex and severe symptomatology. Rather than diagnosing complex presentations as discrete, over-lapping or inter-related co-morbid disorders, I would propose that for many children it is more valid to formulate such complexity as attachment-trauma symptom profiles. These are representations of continuous distributions of symptom types, severity and complexity, which could be referenced to characteristic attachment-trauma symptom clusters identified through research.

A second characteristic of specialised clinical practice with these populations is knowledge and training in the application and interpretation of interview, psychometric and observational measures that are appropriately matched to their particular life circumstances, as well as to the range of mental health difficulties that they manifest. While there are few available population-specific psychometric measures, experienced clinicians in this field tend to conduct quite specialised cross-informant interviews and observations. This aspect of specialised practice is likely to be strengthened over time, as further development and validation of purpose-specific assessment methods unfolds.

A third characteristic pertains to the *comprehensiveness* of clinical assessments. Specialised practice with these populations requires more detailed assessment of attachment- and trauma-related problems, and a wider developmental and contextual focus than that typically employed in mental health clinical assessments. In essence, specialised assessments of these children requires a shift from a relatively narrow, 'mechanical' focus on identifying children's symptoms and disorders – to seeking a comprehensive understanding of children's felt experience, their relationships, family/placement processes, and systemic and care-related influences on children's lives. The case scenario John Simmonds describes in Chapter 11 highlights the critical importance for extending clinical assessments beyond the individual child, to include assessment of the adoptive/foster/kinship family system, and how these systems are influenced by child welfare systemic factors. Clinicians need to enquire about motivations for caregiving and systemic influences on carer roles (Dozier, Grasso, Lindheim, & Lewis, 2007), carer attachment styles (Schofield & Beek, 2005), and carer 'felt security' regarding the permanence of their relationships with the subject child. This is because the primary therapeutic agent for children in care, and those adopted from care, is their substitute family (Schofield & Beek, 2005).

Clinical/psychosocial-developmental scope of practice

The characteristics of specialised clinical practice set out above translate firstly, as increased expertise in the assessment and formulation of attachment- and trauma-related psychopathology among child welfare populations. Secondly, it involves a shift beyond the traditional boundaries of clinical practice to include much greater focus on: the nature of family life that sustains and promotes the development of children who have experienced chronic social adversity; children's felt experiences and world view; child welfare systemic influences; and more detailed consideration of children's developmental histories, with particular reference to attachment and trauma theories. Together this represents a *clinical/psychosocial-developmental* scope of practice that is specific to the development and well-being of child welfare clients, and most particularly to children who are in (or have exited from) alternate care. Clinical/psychosocial-developmental practice is thus as much focused on the minutia of context, as it is with identifying and treating mental health difficulties. It requires the clinician to have a good understanding of age-sensitive psychosocial effects of such things as loss, entry into impermanent care, placement changes, restoration to parental care, length and types of court orders, sibling co-placement, birth family contact, and adoption from care by existing carers versus strangers. It also directs clinicians to enquire about the nature and quality of care that children receive in their present placements, and to learn (where possible) about children's care experiences in previous placements. I believe these factors collectively have greater proximal influence on children's development than do individual clinical interventions. Clinical/psychosocial-developmental practice thus seeks to facilitate therapeutic change and prevent the onset of additional psychopathology, by influencing decisions made by social care agencies, courts and carers. This consultation role is as central to our work as formulation of treatment plans. Clinical/psychosocial-developmental practice also sets out to provide a better platform for conducting psychosocial interventions within the adoptive/foster/kinship family, than standard child clinical practice.

Advocacy

In this section I present a case for *advocacy* being a central component of specialised clinical practice with these children, and most particularly for children and young people with unstable care arrangements. Children in care, and those who have exited care, are some of the most disadvantaged child populations in the western world. Most children enter care following prolonged exposure to harm, during which time there is abject failure of parental responsibility. Once placed in care, many decisions and events that have a bearing on children's well-being are controlled by adults other than their carers. Conversely, foster and kinship carers may be constrained from exercising parental decision-making on such everyday matters as school enrolment, going away on holidays, and having children over for sleepovers. In an ideal world, a child would have one social worker and one set of carers advocating together on his or her behalf, throughout their time in care. Many children who enter care, however, fall well short of gaining this level of support. For some, decisions made for them are compromised by distortions in judgement or empathy, a product of over-burdened or distressed social care agencies. Children in care increasingly encounter high turnover of social workers, resulting in decisions being made by people who have little knowledge of them or their life circumstances. In some jurisdictions, sizeable numbers of children in care have no social worker at all – the so-called unallocated cases. An even more critical factor affecting children's advocacy is placement stability. If a child is raised in a stable adoptive, foster or kinship placement, their carers are better positioned to advocate actively on their behalf. This is because long-term carers tend to have greater knowledge of their children's needs, more established connections with services, and different commitment to children in their long-term care. Children's need for advocacy is not restricted to decision-making within the social care milieu. As described earlier in this chapter, children in care and adopted children can have difficulty accessing mental health and related treatment services, especially if they have complex and severe difficulties that seem resistant to therapeutic change.

Clinicians who specialise in working with children in care should therefore see it as their role to ask 'To what extent is this child or young person alone in the world?' Aside from identifying which people are advocating for a child's needs, specialised clinical practice generates alternative perspectives on what children's needs might be, which can then be used to challenge dominant or prevailing views. At a most human level we need also ask the question 'What would I want for this child, if he or she was *my* child or grandchild?'

Level 2 – service models

This section sets out principles for development of mental health services that support clinical/psychosocial-developmental practice, and which address specific service needs of children in care and those adopted from care.

218 Michael Tarren-Sweeney

Primary – specialist care nexus, and universal assessment

The prevalence, scale and complexity of mental health difficulties experienced by these populations are so great, that delineation between primary and specialist levels of care for these children is blurred. They require universal, comprehensive clinical/psychosocial-developmental assessments following entry into care or adoption. These assessments identify risks and casework-related issues that may contribute to future mental health difficulties, or detract from their development or well-being in other ways. This applies as much to children who enter care with few mental health difficulties. Universal, comprehensive assessment by specialist clinicians following entry into care is thus preferable to mental health screening, because it is designed for prevention of future difficulties as much as detection of present ones. Furthermore, mental health screening alone does not identify critical influences on children's development that have a bearing on other psychosocial-developmental outcomes (that could be remedied if detected early enough). Beyond initial assessment, there remains a need for a primary care (i.e. population-wide) approach to provision of specialist mental health services, equating to a primary – specialist care nexus.

Preventative, long-term engagement and monitoring

Complex attachment- and trauma-related difficulties tend to follow a long developmental course. They are rarely manifested as acute mental health states. In general, the older a child is before they first receive reparative, sensitive care, the more 'trait like' and enduring become their difficulties. Two important goals of mental health interventions with these populations, is to facilitate the development of close relationships, and sustain children's placements. Part of the equation for achieving this is providing carers reliable access to clinical advice and support, so they can be sustained through their most challenging times. Such children and their carers often require ongoing or recurring involvement with mental health services. In these circumstances, continuity of assessment and treatment are important contributors to treatment outcomes. These needs are ill-matched to the predominant 'acute care' focus of public-funded child and adolescent mental health services. Instead, specialised mental health services for these populations should be designed and funded for preventative, long-term engagement and monitoring.

Integral part of social care milieu

In Chapter 9, Kim Golding makes the case for integration between specialist clinical services for adopted and in care children, and social care agencies, citing her experience of multi-agency working in Worcestershire, and an emerging consensus among UK researchers in this field. Golding (2010) describes a number of benefits from service integration, including: an enriched understanding of cases gained through multi-disciplinary problem-solving; the opportunity to carry out coordinated, multi-faceted interventions across different agencies that address a range of related impairments (including mental health); and increased understanding by clinicians of the social context of children's mental health.

Given the present chapter's focus on the development of a clinical specialisation in child welfare work, it is worth re-emphasising the significance of service integration to clinical/psychosocial-developmental practice – namely that such practice *requires* close engagement between mental health and social care services. This is because it provides clinicians greater opportunity to gain understanding of the context of their clients' lives. Social care workplaces are typically intense, stressful and sometimes chaotic. Many services attempt to juggle competing demands and culture of alternate care and child protection teams in the same location. One needs to appreciate the nature of such work to understand how decision-making serves, and occasionally fails children in care. Clinicians who work outside the social care milieu often struggle to comprehend the logic of casework decisions, without understanding constraints imposed on agencies (e.g. a lack of suitable foster placements). Social workers are also often hampered by competing policy guidelines that have very real implications for children's well-being e.g. 'developmental' versus 'natural justice' principles guiding the restoration of children to their birth families. A second reason is that integration facilitates social workers' access to clinical consultation on individual casework. This is very important, given the preventative focus of clinical/psychosocial-developmental practice.

There are various ways of attaining close engagement between mental health and social care services, but each involves some level of integration of clinicians within the social care milieu. To my knowledge there has been no research comparing different integration models. In several Australian states and in New Zealand, statutory agencies operate in-house psychology/psychotherapy services for children who are in their care, as well as for child protection clients and their families. These are either co-located within regional clinical teams, providing services to a number of local offices (as mostly occurs in New Zealand), or work as sole practitioners in front-line social care offices (as mostly occurs in New South Wales). These services work in parallel with CAMHS and other health services i.e. their existence doesn't preclude children from accessing public-funded health services. In many parts of the world, charitable children's agencies also operate in-house psychology/psychotherapy services, sometimes within larger multi-disciplinary health and education teams. A notable example is Casey Family Services in the United States. In Britain, where statutory agencies are much smaller than those in Australasia (operating within local, rather than state or national governments), integration more likely involves some co-location of specialist 'looked after children' CAMHS teams and social care services, or similar multi-agency working through Children's Trusts. A third model sees social care liaison staff located within specialist alternate care CAMHS teams, which can be jointly funded by health and social services departments (Chambers, Saunders, New, Williams, & Stachurska, 2010). Finally, a degree of service integration could be attained using a 'consultation-liaison' model, along similar lines to consultation-liaison psychiatry work in medical wards.

Active ownership

Golding (2010) also describes a number of barriers to mental health services encountered by children and their alternate carers and adoptive parents. Many of these reflect a mismatch between the special circumstances of these populations, and the ways in which generic CAMHS services operate. In some instances, services employ intake criteria that actively block children's access to mental health services, for reasons including the absence of a mental health diagnosis (despite having evident mental health impairment), having the wrong kinds of diagnoses, not having stable placements, not having an identified exit placement, and not gaining access to inpatient care because they are already residing in residential care. It is possible that these situations are not always benign, but in some instances are designed to exclude children who fall into a 'too hard basket'. In addition to reforming referral criteria, these practices can be circumvented if specialist services actively seek to 'own' responsibility for assisting our most challenging children in care.

Normalisation strategies

Balanced against the need for longer-term engagement, and continuity of care through childhood, is perhaps an added potential for causing harm to children or their families. Aside from questions about iatrogenic treatment effects raised earlier in this chapter, we need to consider how long-term engagement with mental health services can become an 'elephant' in children's lives – either by reducing their opportunity for a normalised upbringing (e.g. feeling uncomfortably different from other children), and/or causing distress or anxiety from children's negative perceptions (or experiences) of the service. These risks are not easily mitigated, not least because the training and sensitivities of individual clinicians are likely to have a greater influence on children's perceptions than service models. Notwithstanding this, different approaches to minimising these risks could be implemented at the service level, depending on how much direct involvement is required between children and clinicians. Where there is a need for sustained involvement with children, a useful starting point would be to consider what characteristics of long-term engagement could contribute to children perceiving the service as a source of comfort and reassurance, and as providing some continuity throughout their childhood (especially for those who encounter serial placement changes). For children whose difficulties do not require such direct contact with services, an 'over the horizon' approach to long-term involvement is preferable, with a view to reducing the footprint of service provision on their lives (e.g. delivering interventions via carers, framing our direct contact with children in ways that deflect perceptions of abnormality).

Service alignment

There are potential advantages in aligning specialised mental health services for children in care, those adopted from care and those who return to parental care. Aligning services for these client groups provides greater opportunity for continuity of specialist service delivery through childhood, whether that be for children who proceed from care to adoption, return to their parents' care, or re-enter care following failed restoration or adoption. Secondly, these client groups have similar developmental pathways and mental health patterns. In this regard, children adopted from care have greater affinity with children remaining in care, than with children adopted for other reasons. These client groups are thus similarly matched to the model of specialised clinical practice proposed in this chapter. Thirdly, bearing in mind the high cost of maintaining public-funded specialised mental health services, service alignment provides scope for economic efficiencies.

Balanced against these considerations are some potential drawbacks. The first relates to differences in the level of public funding provided for these groups of children. Where specialised services are funded entirely from health department budgets, then that funding is fairly transparent, and unlikely to lead to differential levels of funding for the different client groups. However, where such services are partly funded by local authorities or children's trusts, there is perhaps greater scope for 'misalignment' of service delivery, such that service access is partly determined by children's legal and care status, rather than their level of need. The second concern is that inequities could arise where there is pressure to accept referrals of children with unstable living arrangements or precarious placements, above other children with similar or greater impairment and distress – a situation that could tilt access away from adopted children.

Civil society

The transfer of parental responsibilities from children's parents to the State involves the transfer of moral as well as legal responsibilities. This extends to ensuring that such children have as much opportunity to flourish, to attain happiness and to form life-sustaining relationships, as we would wish for our own children or grandchildren. Where guardianship rights are later transferred to adoptive parents, the State is presented with another moral imperative – namely, to support those who inherit these parental responsibilities, and who in many instances are burdened with the challenge of raising children with long-term mental ill-health.

Whole of government accountability

In recent years, some governments have resolved that the 'State as parent' is not limited to statutory child welfare agencies, but encompasses all parts of government that can affect the lives of children in care, and by inference, government-funded services. This multi-agency position has emerged partly out of the findings of judicial enquiries into child protection and alternate care systems (Secretary of State for Health & Secretary of State for the Home Department, 2003; Wood, 2008); partly as a consequence of emerging knowledge of ecological influences on children's development that are beyond the reach of child welfare agencies; and partly because of government recognition of the enormous social and economic costs of inter-generational transfer of severe social adversity.

Policies that emphasise a 'whole of government' responsibility for children in care, which is not wholly relinquished when children are subsequently adopted from care, can help reverse the types of discriminatory exclusion practices described earlier in this chapter (particularly in the health and education sectors). Aligned to this is a need to shift away from thinking of the problems of children in care as belonging exclusively to social care agencies. This principle is embodied in the previously mentioned 'Every Child Matters' (Great Britain: Department for Children Schools and Families and Department of Health, 2009) and 'Keep Them Safe' (New South Wales Government, 2010) initiatives, as well as in so-called 'best endeavours' legislation introduced more than a decade ago in New South Wales. The latter provision enables social workers to submit 'best endeavours' requests to other government agencies to provide services that ' ... promote and safeguard the safety, welfare and well-being of a child or young person' ('Children and Young Persons (Care and Protection) Act (NSW)', 1998). Agencies are legally required to make 'best endeavours' to respond to such referrals.

Such legislation is really just the first step in establishing an effective multi-agency response to the mental health and psychosocial needs of these populations. Good policy is critical, but society's responsibility for these children is effectively borne (and interpreted) by individual workers, volunteers and carers. In a recent article, Paula Conway (2009) considers systemic failures in inter-agency working with alternate care and other child welfare clients, characterised by distrust of other agencies and staff, a lack of willingness to cooperate, inadequate communication and blame shifting. Such dysfunctional working relationships are understandable when we consider that they develop among people responding to immensely stressful and distressing situations as part of their everyday work, often without adequate psychological preparation. This can be partly resolved by bringing organisations and individuals together, allowing opportunities for personal connectedness, the communication of shared goals and values, and understanding other agencies' particular challenges and responsibilities. Conway observes, however, that effective relationships often fail to emerge even when opportunities for inter-agency connectedness are mandated through government policy. Bearing in mind the effects of frequent, peripheral exposure to traumatic events and traumatised people, governments need to consider how they can better prepare agencies and their employees for working with children in care and their carers, and with each other.

Note

1 A version of this chapter was previously published as: Tarren-Sweeney, M. (2010). It's time to re-think mental health services for children in care, and those adopted from care. *Clinical Child Psychology and Psychiatry*, 15(4), 613–626.

References

Bellamy, J., Traube, D., & Gopalan, G. (2010). 'A national study of the impact of outpatient mental health services for children in long-term foster care'. *Clinical Child Psychology and Psychiatry*, 15(4), 467–480.

Chambers, M., Saunders, A., New, B., Williams, C., & Stachurska, A. (2010). 'Assessment of children coming into care: Processes, pitfalls and partnerships'. *Clinical Child Psychology and Psychiatry*, 15(4), 511–527.

Children and Young Persons (Care and Protection) Act (NSW)(1998).

Cicchetti, D., Toth, S. L., & Maughan, A. (2000). 'An ecological-transactional model of child maltreatment'. In A. Sameroff & M. Lewis (Eds.), *Handbook of developmental psychopathology (2nd ed.)* (pp. 689–722). Dordrecht, Netherlands: Kluwer Academic Publishers.

Conway, P. (2009). 'Falling between minds: The effects of unbearable experiences on multi-agency communication in the care system'. *Adoption & Fostering*, 33(1), 18–28.

Crittenden, P. M. (1997). 'Toward an integrative theory of trauma: A dynamic-maturation approach'. In D. Cicchetti & S. L. Toth (Eds.), *Developmental perspectives on trauma: Theory, research, and intervention. Rochester symposium on developmental psychology*, Vol. 8 (pp. 33–84). Rochester, NY: University of Rochester Press.

DeJong, M. (2010). 'Some reflections on the use of psychiatric diagnosis in the looked after or "in care" child population'. *Clinical Child Psychology & Psychiatry*, 15(4), 589–599.

Dozier, M., Grasso, D., Lindheim, O., & Lewis, E. (2007). 'The role of caregiver committment in foster care: Insights from the This Is My Baby Interview'. In D. Oppenheim & D. Goldsmith (Eds.), *Attachment theory in clinical work with children: Bridging the gap between research and practice* (pp. 90–108). New York: Guilford Press.

Fonagy, P., & Bateman, A. (2006). 'Progress in the treatment of borderline personality disorder'. *British Journal of Psychiatry*, 188, 1–3.

Golding, K. (2010). 'Multi-agency and specialist working to meet the mental health needs of children in care and adopted'. *Clinical Child Psychology and Psychiatry*, 15(4), 573–587.

Great Britain: Department for Children Schools and Families and Department of Health. (2008). *Response to children and young people in mind: Final report of the national CAMHS review*. London, Great Britain: Department for Children, Schools and Families and Department of Health.

Great Britain: Department for Children Schools and Families and Department of Health. (2009). *Statutory guidance on promoting the health and well-being of looked after children*. London, Great Britain: Department for Children, Schools and Families and Department of Health.

Kreppner, J., O'Connor, T., Rutter, M., Beckett, C., Castle, J., Croft, C., et al. (2001). 'Can inattention / overactivity be an institutional deprivation syndrome?'. *Journal of Abnormal Child Psychology, 29*(6), 513–528.

Landsverk, J., Burns, B., Stambaugh, L., & Reutz, J. (2009). 'Psychosocial interventions for children and adolescents in foster care: Review of research literature'. *Child Welfare, 88*(1), 49–69.

Leslie, L., Hurlburt, M., James, S., Landsverk, J., Slymen, D. J., & Zhang, J. (2005). 'Relationship between entry into child welfare and mental health service use'. *Psychiatric Services, 56*(8), 981–987.

Leslie, L., Kelleher, K., Burns, B., Landsverk, J., & Rolls, J. (2003). 'Foster care and Medicaid managed care'. *Child Welfare, 82*(3), 367–392.

National Institute for Clinical Excellence NICE. (2005). '*Depression in children and young people' Clinical Guidelines CG28*. United Kingdom: The British Psychological Society.

New South Wales Government. (2010). *Keep them safe: A shared approach to child wellbeing*. Retrieved April 2010, from http://www.keepthemsafe.nsw.gov.au/home

O'Connor, T., & Zeanah, C. (2003). 'Current perspectives on attachment disorders: Rejoinder and synthesis'. *Attachment and Human Development, 5*(3), 321–326.

Romanelli, L., Landsverk, J., Levitt, J., Leslie, L. K., Hurley, M., Bellonci, C., et al. (2009). 'Best practices for mental health in child welfare: Screening, assessment, and treatment guidelines'. *Child Welfare, 88*(1), 163–188.

Royal Australian & New Zealand College of Psychiatrists. (2008). *The mental health care needs of children in out-of-home care: A report from the expert working committee of the Faculty of Child and Adolescent Psychiatry*. Melbourne: RANZCP.

Schofield, G., & Beek, M. (2005). 'Providing a secure base: Parenting children in long-term foster family care'. *Attachment and Human Development, 7*(1), 3–25.

Secretary of State for Health, & Secretary of State for the Home Department (Writer). (2003). *The Victoria Climbié inquiry: Report of an inquiry by Lord Laming*. London: HMSO.

Sturgess, W., & Selwyn, J. (2007). 'Supporting the placements of children adopted out of care'. *Clinical Child Psychology and Psychiatry, 12*(1), 13–28.

Tarren-Sweeney, M. (2008). 'The mental health of children in out-of-home care'. *Current Opinion in Psychiatry, 21*, 345–349.

Tarren-Sweeney, M. (In Press). 'An investigation of complex attachment- and trauma-related symptomatology among children in foster and kinship care'. *Child Psychiatry and Human Development*. Online first, DOI: 10.1007/s10578-013-0366-x.

van der Kolk, B. (2005). 'Developmental trauma disorder'. *Psychiatric Annals, 35*(5), 401–408.

Wood, J. (2008). *Report of the special commission of inquiry into child protection services in NSW (the Wood report)*. Sydney: NSW Government.

Index

access to mental health services for adoptive families, 166
active responsibility for care populations, 220
Adult Attachment Interview, 122, 131
advocacy role for clinicians, 155, 217
age at entry into care, 6
aligning services to include adopted children, 166, 221
Assessment Checklist for Children, 12, 189
attachment, 5, 6, 88, 100, 101, 119–20, 123, 125–34, 185–87
Attachment and Biobehavioral Catchup, 39, 44, 53, 79
attachment difficulties, 12, 185–87
Attachment Narrative Therapy, 39, 125–36
attachment-based assessment, 88, 92
availability of mental health services, 14

background to alternate care and adoption systems, 4–5, 85, 100
barriers to accessing mental health services, 165–67
birth family contact, 100

California Evidence-based Clearinghouse for Child Welfare treatment ratings, 41, 154
CAMHS service models for children in care, 86, 154, 141–57, 170, 189, 198, 219
capacity of mental health services, 211
caregiver attachment histories, 122–23
caregiver interventions, 39, 63
carer-child observations, 107
characteristic mental health difficulties of children in care, 12, 151, 162, 183–85
Child-Parent Psychotherapy, 45
children adopted from care, 61
clinical practice guidelines, 40, 204, 206
clinical treatment trials, 41, 47–55, 61–80
clinical/psychosocial-developmental scope of practice, 205, 213, 216

clinically meaningful treatment effectiveness, 49
clinician skill and training, 94, 215
cognitive behavioural interventions, 63
complex psychopathology, 13, 38, 51, 151, 152, 162, 189, 212, 218
complex trauma, 151, 187, 189
comprehensiveness of clinical assessments, 215
concurrent planning, 54, 86, 89
consultation-liaison model, 220
costs of treatment, 52, 65, 71, 122
cumulative adversity, 6

development and causes of mental ill-health, 5–9, 163, 181
developmental pathways, 5
Developmental Trauma Disorder, 188
Dialectical Behaviour Therapy, 38, 39, 46
Dyadic Developmental Psychotherapy, 39, 78

early intervention, 87, 99, 171
effectiveness of mental health interventions, 28–33, 37–55, 142, 212
effects of maltreatment, 5, 7, 8, 10, 87, 99
emotional needs of children in care and adopted children, 120
Enhanced Adoptive Parenting, 39, 61–80, 199
evaluating psychotherapy effectiveness, 47, 55, 74
evidence hierarchy, 47
evidence-based interventions, 37, 198, 212
evidence-based practice, 40, 46–48
exclusionary policies, 170

family behavioural interventions, 39
family therapy, 39, 153
felt security, 3, 5, 7, 45, 54, 55, 142, 153

government initiatives for mental health service delivery, 210, 222
group psychotherapy, 38

harmful treatment effects, 52, 149, 213

inadequacy of acute care service model, 211, 218
indigenous and ethnic minority children in care and adopted, 4, 23, 46, 53
individual psychotherapy, 38
influences on mental health service use, 23–24
integration of mental health and social care services, 163, 161–75, 218–20

KEEP intervention, 44, 77, 79, 199

long-term engagement by mental health services, 218
loss, 5, 132, 151, 194

mandatory health assessment, 101, 103
mental health assessment measures, 11, 12, 13, 64, 106
mental health of children adopted from care, 12, 62, 162
mental health of children in care and adopted children, 10, 11–13, 84, 100, 161, 195
mental health of children in kinship care, 11
mental health of children in residential care, 11, 84
mental health service models, 86, 141–57, 189, 217
mentalisation-based treatment, 39
multi-agency working, 145, 146, 147, 148, 154, 163, 161–75, 190, 218–20
Multidimensional Treatment Foster Care, 39, 42, 199
Multidimensional Treatment Foster Care for Preschoolers, 39, 42–43, 53, 79
multiple evidence requirements, 48
multi-systemic interventions, 39, 171

New Orleans intervention, 95
NICE/SCIE public health guidelines, 41, 102, 198
normalisation strategies, 220
nosological quandaries, 183–85
NSCAW – National Survey of Child and Adolescent Well-being, 24, 37, 212

Parent Child Interaction Therapy, 39, 153
Parent-Child Psychotherapy, 39
parenting measures, 68

patterns of mental health service use, 13–16, 22–23, 100
permanency, 7, 86, 88, 100, 102
placement instability, 7, 85, 88, 101
play therapy, 38
pre-natal influences, 181
prevention of mental ill-health, 38, 87, 171, 218
primary-specialist care nexus, 218
profile approach to clinical formulation, 215

RANZCP practice guidelines, 41
rates of children in care and adopted children, 4
Reactive Attachment Disorder, 151, 185–87
referral process, 148
reviews of mental health treatments, 40

screening, 116, 218
sculpting technique, 133
sexual abuse counselling, 38
social deficits, 185
social workers as therapists, 9
specialised assessment, 150, 169
specialised clinical practice, 204, 205, 213, 214
specialised mental health services, 163
specialist mental health services, 101, 141–57, 213
specificity of mental health interventions, 39
sub-threshold presentations, 182
systemic context of growing up in care, 154, 165, 197–99, 207, 215, 216, 219
systemic therapy, 39

trauma, 132, 142, 151, 187–89
Trauma-focussed CBT, 38, 45
treatment effectiveness outcome measures, 51, 74
types of alternate care and adoption, 4–5
types of mental health treatment, 38, 152

under-referral of children in care to mental health services, 101, 165
universal comprehensive assessment, 204, 218
universal screening, 102, 204, 211

validity of diagnostic classification systems, 13, 51, 151, 180–90, 212
vicarious traumatisation of clinicians, 155
views of children and young people in care, 165

whole of government accountability, 222